GOOD GENES GONE BAD

ADVANCE PRAISE FOR THE BOOK

'This is a wonderful and highly educational book written in breezy but scientifically accurate prose. The stories and characters in the book make medicine, and the science behind it, come alive. It is a must-read for anyone interested in medicine or biology'—Siddhartha Mukherjee, author, *The Emperor of All Maladies: A Biography of Cancer* and *The Gene: An Intimate History*, and associate professor, Columbia University

'We all wish that the development of new therapies could be straight, level and fast. But, as Naren illustrates so well, the road is almost always full of twists and turns, hills and valleys, that must be navigated with both patience and ingenuity'—Bruce Levine, Barbara and Edward Netter professor, Cancer Gene Therapy, University of Pennsylvania, Philadelphia

'*Good Genes Gone Bad* presents the vast developmental scenario of biologics, connecting numerous path-breaking researches of yore with successfully marketed drugs. He is one of that rare breed of scientists who are blessed with the ability to present complex issues like a storyteller to the general public. The book also presents a glimpse into the functioning and strengths of Biocon, a major biologics Indian pharma. The book is a delight to read and I personally single out two chapters, "An Elusive Vaccine to Prevent AIDS" and "The Story of Immunotherapy", for their ability to emphasize the complex, high-risk and uncertain nature of new drug discovery. With the ongoing COVID-19 pandemic, there is a public need to demystify and understand immunology, and this book makes it pleasurable to learn. I strongly and wholeheartedly recommend the book as a must-read for biomedical researchers and also for science enthusiasts'—Madhu Dikshit, ex-director, Central Drug Research Institute, Lucknow

'The ability to stitch a story from the most sordid moments in history to eureka-like ones is really Naren's in the making. I find Naren's prose to be a fitting coming together of facts, learning and lore in the space of biology and drug development. His ability to tell a story with lucidity and reverence is what really sets it apart. Thanks for telling our collective stories through your wisdom'—Kavitha Iyer-Rodrigues, CEO, Zumutor Biologics Inc., Bangalore

GOOD GENES GONE BAD

A SHORT HISTORY OF VACCINES AND BIOLOGICS: FAILURES, SUCCESSES, CONTROVERSIES

NARENDRA CHIRMULE

EBURY
PRESS

An imprint of Penguin Random House

EBURY PRESS

USA | Canada | UK | Ireland | Australia
New Zealand | India | South Africa | China

Ebury Press is part of the Penguin Random House group of companies
whose addresses can be found at global.penguinrandomhouse.com

Published by Penguin Random House India Pvt. Ltd
4th Floor, Capital Tower 1, MG Road,
Gurugram 122 002, Haryana, India

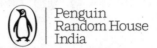

Penguin
Random House
India

First published in Ebury Press by Penguin Random House India 2021

ISBN 9780670096039

Typeset in Sabon by Manipal Technologies Limited, Manipal
Printed at Replika Press Pvt. Ltd, India

www.penguin.co.in

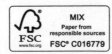

MIX
Paper from
responsible sources
FSC® C016779

To Anisha and Lin,
who have taught me about courage

Contents

Foreword

I am delighted that Naren has chosen to write a whole book on failures in drug development. Whilst it is well acknowledged that high failure rates are part and parcel of the high-risk, high-reward lab to market journey of drugs, no one has shone the spotlight on this inherent but often underestimated challenge. I have had my share of failures along my entrepreneurial journey and I know that drug development is certainly not for the faint-hearted! However, I have also learnt that success does eventually emerge from overcoming challenges, leading with conviction and following the science.

There is a desperate need to improve and enhance the processes of drug development. New technologies and advanced biological and computational science can surely provide us ways to accelerate regulatory processes that seek strong safety and efficacy signals for approval. The COVID-19 pandemic has shown us that drugs and vaccines can be developed in a very short span of time, where there is urgency. There has also been an unprecedented level of collaboration, information sharing and a common sense of purpose. It need not have taken a pandemic to shine the light on these obvious factors of success but as the adage goes 'it's better late than never'. The pharmaceutical industry, if I may say so, is engrossed in getting ahead of competition and often loses sight of the true-north, which is to develop drugs for patients no matter where they live or whether they are rich or poor. Political and cultural differences, economic requirements, and priorities of societal needs in different regions of the world influence the decisions for access and advances to healthcare. The skewed focus on investing in non-communicable diseases, to the detriment of underinvesting in infectious diseases, has exposed the dangerous vulnerability of human beings to invisible microbes. The pandemic is an inflection point for the pharmaceutical and biotechnology industry to reevaluate the processes of drug development systematically and to focus on health equity as the economic purpose.

When I embarked on my entrepreneurial journey of building Biocon in 1978, I did not have the faintest idea that it would be a multibillion-dollar company with nearly 20,000 employees. With various stops and starts along the way, I was supported by many mentors, advisers, well-wishers, all of whom played a vital role in realizing my goals. Four decades later, I am still driven by a deep sense of purpose to transform access to essential and life-saving medicines to patients who are in need anywhere in the world.

Naren joined the Biocon leadership team as Head of R&D in 2015 and bought into this ethos of affordable access. Under his leadership, Biocon saw the global approval of biosimilar trastuzumab and glargine which delivered on our stated goal of affordable innovation. With the experience he has garnered from the companies he previously worked in such as Merck and Amgen, and the experiences he gained in Biocon, he is well placed to do a systematic analysis of the multi-factorial elements in the development of biologics and vaccines.

This book is a summary of not just the science of the drugs developed for the treatment of some difficult-to-treat diseases, but also a personal story of his view of the failures involved in drug development, from which he has listed several lessons. This book will be valuable for all practitioners of drug development, and students who will follow their dreams in researching new drugs. The simplicity of the language makes it amenable for the general public to understand the trials and tribulations involved in drug development.

Kiran Mazumdar-Shaw,
executive chairperson,
Biocon Limited

Prologue

Who am I?

In 2019, I attended a writing class aptly named 'Bangalore's World-Famous Semi-Deluxe Writing Programme'. As pre-work for the class, we were given an assignment to write an essay on 'Who am I'.

A profound statement that can be interpreted in so many ways: from a simple, 'I am Narendra Chirmule', to Ramana Maharshi's thought-provoking process of deep introspection. I will explore this statement through a letter to myself.

It is 1977. You have just moved from a wonderful school experience full of great friends and living in a protected railway colony of Research Design Standards Organization (RDSO), where your father worked, in Lucknow to Bombay. Seven has been your lucky number, so starting college, at Ramniranjan Jhunjhunwala College,

*on 7-7-77 was quite fortuitous. You had no specific idea
of what you wanted to do and be (and that is totally
fine!). You liked chemistry and biology, but mathematics
and physics, not so much. That was not because of the
Chemistry and Biology subjects, but because of the teachers
who taught those subjects in school. Drs Ajoy Gon and
A.U. Khan influenced the subjects more because of their
teaching styles. You really liked English but knew that just
English would not make a career. Hindi was just another
language you had to learn, but you got more than your
share of it by living in Lucknow; you will appreciate it
later in life for many reasons, not the least of them being
the ability to talk to ministers in Delhi making big policy
decisions. You should take more interest in reading and
writing since these are lifelong friends (Appa's favourite
rhyme was 'my never-failing friends are they, with whom
I converse day-by-day'). Every subject you (did not) learn
will be important for the future. For example, statistics, a
very uninteresting subject now, will be invaluable in your
job in the future; economics will be fascinating as you make
your own money, and how the environment (political,
ecological, cultural) influences it, not to mention history
and geography.*

*Moving to Bombay from a small town, where you were
living in a protected environment, was a culture shock.
Vinay Madan, your friend in college, made it much easier
to assimilate into the culture. After earning your master's
in zoology you did your PhD in applied biology on the*

development of an anti-leprosy vaccine.* Studying leprosy was your first lesson in immunology, as the disease spans a wide spectrum of both cell-mediated and humoral immune responses. A lesson learnt during this time was that earning a PhD is a process of learning the method and process of conducting scientific research and solving extremely difficult problems, and the subject is just the means to do it. Many PhD students put too much focus on the subject.

The PhD exercise was long and tough work, or so you thought at that time. It was also very physical, since you had to go to Acworth Leprosy Hospital every day to pick up samples, and to Satpati to monitor the clinical trial. Thanks to your bicycle, you were very mobile. It was also a good way to get exercise, in the days when workouts and gyms were not in fashion, especially in India. You learnt the basics of immunology. Although the assays you used were ancient (SRBC rosettes, ox-RBC rosettes, ELISA), the biology (nay, biotechnology) you were involved with in developing a sub-unit vaccine for leprosy was way ahead of its time. Rita Mulherkar, a senior scientist at Cancer Research Institute, who had received her training in Budapest, Hungary, had an enormous influence on your way of thinking about immunology. Dr Madhav Deo was your PhD guide. An extremely thoughtful scientist who always thought out of the box, and was your idol.

---

* Jayaraman, K.S. 'India Carries Out Large-Scale Tests of Anti-Leprosy Vaccine'. *Nature* 328 (1987): 660.

There was also much non-science you learnt while studying science: i) the art of negotiation with peers and your superiors; ii) the value of networking; iii) how to make good friends at work that you could trust; iv) collaboration; v) getting things done; vi) the importance of verbal, written and unspoken communication; and importantly vii) having fun while doing intense and important work. What you did not have was a true mentor; someone who showed you direction in life, a 'sat-guru'. This person, you did not have even in later years.

Your post-doctoral research in the pathogenesis of AIDS at North Shore University Hospital–Cornell University Medical College, New York, shaped and established the foundation of your knowledge of immunology. The ten-year period from 1985 to 1995 saw an explosion in the field of immuno-virology,* and the team you worked with contributed to this body of work through several key publications. Understanding the mechanism of the pathogenesis of the severe immune suppression in HIV-infected individuals involved an in-depth study of the multi-component dysfunction of the immune system.

In 1996, you were appointed as a faculty member at the University of Pennsylvania, Philadelphia, in the Department of Medicine and Institute for Human Gene Therapy. The original research work done in the therapy

---

* Pillars in Immunology. https://www.jimmunol.org/pillarsofimmunology. (Last accessed on 14 May 2021).

of genetic diseases using viral vectors resulted in significant publications, which have been extensively cited. The retrospective study of the pathogenesis of the severe adverse events associated with adenoviral vectors provided clues to the development of a safer and more efficacious adeno-associated viral vector. These studies on new viral vectors have transformed the field of gene therapy, yielding successful therapies for a few monogenic diseases.

You then joined Merck in 2000, located in the West Point campus near Philadelphia, as director of the department of vaccines and biologics. You were responsible for the development and implementation of assays for measuring immune responses to vaccines. Key among these vaccines were Gardasil® (human papillomavirus), RotaTeq® (rotavirus) and Zostavax® (varicella), which were granted global regulatory approvals. Gardasil® vaccine prevents HPV-induced cervical cancer; RotaTeq® vaccine prevents rotavirus-induced gastroenteritis, dehydration and death in children; and Zostavax® vaccine prevents development of shingles caused by the chicken-pox virus, varicella zoster. You also worked on the development of the adenovirus vector-based HIV vaccine, which was tested in the seminal STEP trial. The clinical trial is a landmark study which evaluated the potential efficacy of the HIV vaccines. The study failed, and failed badly. The results of the trial were instrumental in informing the field of HIV vaccines on the importance of both cell as well as humoral immune protective immune responses. Thanks to your work in this area, you were appointed to the NIH study section committee for HIV, which is a group of ten scientists, with diverse experiences. The committee reviews grant proposals and provides recommendations for funding innovative ideas for developing novel HIV vaccines.

In 2007, you joined Amgen, based in California, as executive director of the department of clinical immunology. In this role, you contributed extensively to the white papers and regulatory guidances in the immunogenicity of biologics, publishing extensively on novel methodologies of measuring immune responses to biologics, the utilization of quality-by-design approaches of molecule design, and statistical methods for analyses of the pharmacokinetic and pharmacodynamics of biologics.

In 2014, your Amgen days came to end. This was partly your choice, and partly not. You would have been comfortable continuing to enjoy the luxuries of life that Amgen provided. A big home. A fancy car. A good friends circle. The utopian environment of Thousand Oaks. But it was not to be. It had been seven years, and typically you get restless after this time period. You gave serious thought to moving to India. There were several pros and cons to consider. Ravi Khare, who is your friend from teenage years, your brother-in-law, and now business partner, was very objective in his advice. He is probably someone who knows you the best. His advice was based on his own experiences in doing business in the Indian environment and in thirty other countries. He highlighted dishonesty, egoism and sycophancy, a lack of commitment to anything, the lack of a scientific approach and a haphazard way of doing things (jugaad), among many other cons. You added some more to this list. Corruption, social inequality, lack of cleanliness, politics. On the pros. i) Your daughter, Anisha is very happy and settled with her partner, Lin, in Philadelphia, hence you had no major immediate family responsibility and engagements; ii) the science being done in Biocon was of the highest international standards; iii) the scientists you had met were extremely knowledgeable; iv) management at Biocon was eager for transformative changes; and v) you were eager to spend time in India to be with family there. Bangalore was the obvious choice since your sister, Anjali Rao, lived there. The opportunity to contribute to the development of biologics and support the team to obtain regulatory approval, in a leadership role, was very exciting and challenging. You would have the freedom to share your experiences and put new processes in place to develop a culture of an organization.

2015 and beyond. As head of research and development (R&D) at Biocon Research Labs in Bangalore, you were responsible for developing the pipeline of novel biologics and biosimilars. Biologics are a new class of drugs that are made from living things, e.g. human proteins made in bacteria. Biosimilars are the generic versions of biologics, after their patent has expired. R&D at Biocon comprised the chevron of processes, ranging cell line engineering, upstream and downstream process development of drug substance and drug product, toxicology, physico-chemical and bio-analytical, clinical trials, regulatory and intellectual property groups. During your three-plus-year tenure at Biocon, which was one of the most satisfying experiences of your career, the company got regulatory approvals for trastuzumab biosimilar for treatment of breast cancer and glargine for the treatment diabetes.

You were fifty-eight. It was time to retire from the corporate world.

It was then that you started your entrepreneurial journey. With your friend and confidant, Ravi Khare, you established SymphonyTech Biologics, a data analytics company that explores the space between mathematics and biology. Its tag line is 'finding engineering solutions to biological problems'. It's been two years now since retirement, and time to write your book.

Why this book?

My experiences in drug development in the various places I worked in during the course of my career took me through several failures. Colossal failures. In all cases, these failures were followed by phenomenal successes. Indeed, were it not for the failures, the paths to success that followed would have been hazy, long-winding and tiresome. To appreciate success, it is important to chronicle and recognize the contribution of the things that went wrong. The process of drug development needs a seismic change. The COVID-19 pandemic has highlighted the possibility of developing safe and effective drugs and vaccines in unprecedented timelines. The data from the lessons learnt from these processes need to be collected, analysed, and applied to all drug development in the pharmaceutical and biotechnology industries. Hence this book.

As I embarked on writing this book, several reasons for doing so emerged through the course of the exercise. I wanted to share my experiences in drug development; collate the collective experience of all my colleagues who have contributed to the development of these drugs; understand the complexity and magnitude of the nature of work required to get drugs approved; provide an understanding of the risks during drug development and lay out a process to plan for mitigating them; determine the factors for success and failure; share the personal face of drug development through the people in the pharmaceutical industry; and create awareness that it is a collaboration of industry, academia, government and society (patients, caregivers, investors, etc.) that develops medicines which help create novel drugs for human health.

I hope the stories I have narrated provide readers with a sense of the magnitude of the challenges and the extent of the difficulty in making novel medicines. Each drug has a unique path, which is riddled with challenges. The general public is unaware of the complexity of the drug development process. In fact, the entire process is not known even to insiders in academia and industry. It was not until I had more than fifteen years of experience in the industry that I gained a true understanding of the multi-disciplinary nature of drug development. Hence the stories I have chosen are remarkable for the perseverance of the people behind the drug, which has made it possible for us (the patient) to get innovative treatments for diseases. I am grateful to the hundreds of colleagues I have worked with over the years who have shared their experiences. The collaborative process has been extremely rewarding.

The narration of this book follows a pattern. I love the number seven. It is my date of birth in January; my first day of college was on 7-7-77; there are seven days in a week; there is a seven-beat rhythm (taal) in tabla (*rupak*); there are seven continents, seven seas and seven colours of the rainbow. The lists I make in the book have seven points. There are seven stories I have chosen to tell. But why seven? Why not, I say? Making a list of seven requires effort. It is very easy to make a list of three things. Try making a list of seven for everything; you have to think hard and deep.

I have also used analogies, which I find are an interesting way to explain the complexities of biological systems, to help readers understand a concept.

The process of narration is interspersed with questions. It is often difficult to be able to ask the right questions in any given situation. These days it is quite easy to find answers

to anything and everything by Googling. However, since it is critical to learn how to ask insightful questions, I have listed below a process that will help in doing so.

There are four levels of distinct understanding:

1) Data, which comes in many forms, shapes and sizes and needs to be organized.
2) Information, which is derived from an analysis of data.
3) Knowledge, which arises from information once it is processed.
4) Wisdom, which emerges from an assimilation of orthogonal knowledge.

The journey from one level to the next can be made by asking relevant questions.

Data → Information
Questions generally start with what, when, where, who (when did you buy this shirt?).

Information → Knowledge
Questions generally start with how (how did you buy this shirt?).

To illustrate, if one considers each subject, anatomy, physiology, biochemistry, etc., to be an individual piece of information, then when combined, one has the knowledge of medicine.

Knowledge → Wisdom
Questions generally start with why (why did you wear this shirt?). These questions often require a philosophical answer.

To illustrate, the knowledge of medicine, combined with people skills, communication skills and emotional intelligence, makes one 'wise'.

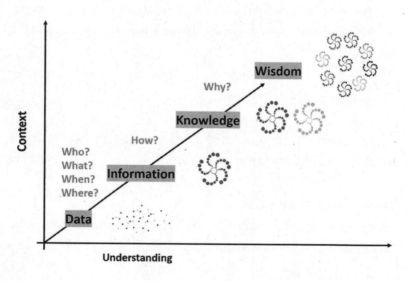

The stories I have chosen to narrate follow a specific pattern: i) the inception of an excellent idea to change the course of a treatment paradigm of a disease; ii) the process of drug development in that study; iii) the failure that resulted; iv) the lessons learnt; v) a new ideation that resulted (inflection point); vi) the development of the new idea (based on the learnings); and vii) the success story.

	I Haemophilia: a genetic disorder for which we are close to finding a cure	II Rotavirus vaccine: a story of courage and faith in developing a vaccine that saved millions of lives	III HIV vaccine: one of the most challenging vaccines, it is yet to be developed by mankind	IV Cancer immunotherapy: a revolution in the cure of cancer	V Cell therapy: the story of persistence, extreme focus and dedication, which has changed the field of medicine	VI Gene therapy: the trials and tribulations on the path towards the final frontier of medicine	VII Biocon story
1 The initial idea	Blood transfusion	Rhesus rotavirus vaccine	gp120 neutralizing antibody	TGN1412 (anti-CD28)	SCID Severe Combined Immune Deficiency patients	Adenovirus vector	
2 Development	Trial	Trial	Trial	Preclinical and clinical trials	Lentivirus vector	Preclinical studies and initial clinical success	
3 Failure	AIDS	Intussusception	Failed	Severe Adverse Events (SAE) in healthy subjects Cytokine Storm Syndrome (CRS)	SAE, caused leukaemia	SAE, death	

#							
4	Lessons	Diagnosis	Rare SAE	HIV is highly variable	Super-activation of immune system	Understanding how to develop safe vectors	Understanding of inflammation	
5	New idea INFLECTION POINT	Recombinant factors	Bovine vaccine (RotaTeq)	CD8 T cell	ipi/pembro	Chimeric Antigen Receptor T cells (CAR-T cell) therapy	AAV vector (Luxterna)	
6	Development	Trial	Very large trial	Trial failed again	Phase 1/2	Long clinical trials	Long preclinical trial; small clinical trial	
7	Success	Approval	Approval	New idea	Approval (cure)	Approval of CAR-T cells	Approval	First biologic approved in the US and EU
	Next phase	+Novel drug	Global access	Trial underway	Many checkpoint inhibitor trials	Cancer cure	Hemlibra novel treatment	

As you will see, all stories follow a pattern of a colossal failure, an inflection point, followed by a revolutionary discovery or invention that transforms the treatment of that disease.

Thus the flow in the chapters reads as follows:

Chapter 1 The Story of Haemophilia:

i) the use of normal human serum to treat the disease; ii) the temporary success for patients; iii) the advent of AIDS; iv) the plan to develop a recombinant product (*inflection point*); v) the design of the new class of clotting factors (*inflection point*); vi) clinical trials; and vii) approval and success for patients.

Chapter 2 The Rotavirus Vaccine:

i) the novel idea of molecular combination of rhesus and human rotaviruses (called reassortants) to design a vaccine; ii) the clinical trials; iii) deaths due to a rare side effect: intussusception (blocking of the intestine due to telescopic folding); iv) the design of a new reassortant with bovine rotavirus (*inflection point*); v) planning the criteria for clinical trials; vi) conducting a very large clinical trial; and vii) success and a major impact in terms of saving children from dying.

as the inhibitory pathway (*inflection point*); v) the design of plans for the clinical trials and end points; vi) clinical trials; and vii) success of ipilimumab and pembrolizumab in treatment of previously untreatable cancers such as melanoma.

Chapter 6 The Story of Gene Therapy:

i) Bone Marrow Transplantation (BMT) to treat immunological diseases such as severe combined immune-deficiency (SCID) gene therapies, and evolution of gene therapy to modify the bone-marrow cells with vectors (modified viruses which transport genes) e.g., lentiviruses; ii) clinical trials; iii) unanticipated induction of leukaemia; iv) plans for CAR-T cells which involve development of processes to take cells from a patient, transform them into killer T cells, and re-infuse them back into the patients (*inflection point*); v) design of the clinical trials and clinical end points; vi) execution of clinical trials and regulatory approval; and vii) success in treatment of patients with various types of leukemias.

Chapter 7 Biocon and My Own Story of Biotechnology:

i) History of biotechnology, ii) history of Biocon, iii) people in Biocon; iv) landmark regulatory approvals v) plans for preparing for approval of trastuzumab biosimilar for the treatment of breast cancer; vi) executing the plan from manufacturing to clinical trials, and vii) success of the approval process

The COVID-19 Chapter:

i) COVID-19 arrives; ii) early learnings; iii) the first wave, India is not in it; iv) vaccine are being developed; v) vaccines are approved; vi) the success of vaccinations; vii) the second wave and beyond.

Inflection points:

An inflection point is the point in the curve of a graph where the shape changes. Instead of continuing on a linear path, it changes direction. The reasons for the change can be attributed to several factors that occurred before the inflection point.

INFLECTION POINT IS ALWAYS BEHIND YOU

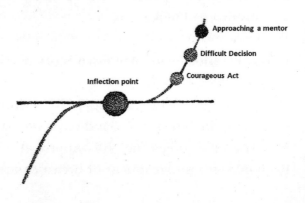

An illustrative example is that of a cell culture. When cells are growing in a culture flask in a laboratory, they are 'happy' because of the following reasons: i) abundant fresh media; ii) a good environment of oxygen, appropriate temperature and pH; iii) genetically appropriate conditions for replication and proliferation; iv) presence of growth factors; v) plenty of space; vi) no competition; and vii) overall healthy conditions. All these factors orchestrate the exponential growth of cells in the culture flask. Then the inflection point appears, and the shape of the curve changes.

After a few days of the culture, the cells stop growing; in fact, they start dying, for the following reasons: i) the resources of media are exhausted; ii) carbon dioxide, ammonia, methane and a low pH have made the environment inhospitable; iii) genetically the cells are exhausted; iv) the cells start secreting toxins; v) space is limited; vi) there is now a lot of competition; and vii) overall the conditions are unhealthy. Another inflection point appears, and the cells start dying.

Another example is one's career. Factors that influence the inflection of a career curve can include courage, respect, discipline, attitude/passion, effective communication, truthfulness and health.

The stories in this book involve studies of biological drugs, vaccines, cell therapy and finally gene therapy: the holy grail of medicine, to correct and cure a disease at its root. It is not just fantasy. Major advances have been made to realize the potential of this human endeavour. Glimmers of success are now being observed. Rare diseases, primarily with single gene defects, are being 'cured'. The learning process of humans (sometimes called innovation) is something that is eternal and persistent. Discovery and inventions are an integral part of the human psyche. Continuous improvement over what we have is the mantra; sometimes incremental and sometimes exponential.

Innovation:

Innovation is required for solving problems. Difficult problems. If the problem is considered to be a box, then the process to solve it involves breaking the box into smaller manageable parts (problems) and solving each one separately. Once all the smaller boxes are considered solved, the larger box is reconstructed to determine whether the original problem was solved. Usually in this process, one of the smaller boxes (problems) was so difficult that it was not really solved. Yet, when the larger box is reconstructed, we squint our eyes and assume and conclude that the larger problem is solved. Alas, frequently, the problem solved with this approach does not stand the test of time, and the box (problem) eventually falls apart. This process of innovation is the 'top-down' approach. Many examples of medicines, such as Vioxx by Merck, which underwent extensive clinical trials but failed due to cardiovascular side effects, are case studies for this approach to innovation.

The 'bottom-up' approach to innovation is used by Nature. All the 'problems' that Nature must solve are extremely difficult ones. A tadpole must develop legs and lungs through a process of evolution before it can emerge out of water as a frog and survive on land. This innovation by Nature involves trial and error of many different gene mutations, which create tadpole parts, which must undergo the process of survival of the fittest. Until the lungs and feet of the frog evolved, it could not walk on land. This process of innovation requires small but incremental changes, a lot of resources, time and patience. But, once the innovation solution is achieved, it lasts forever.

THE JOURNEY OF INNOVATION

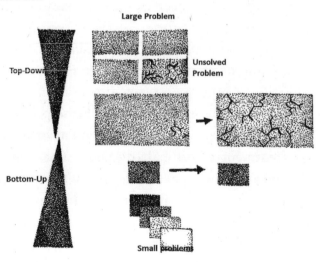

Innovation in biotechnology can also be approached by the top-down and bottom-up approaches. The stories of success (the frog) evolve through systematically solving each problem (tadpole). Each failure is a stepping stone to success. This process is a testament to the perseverance of mankind. The stories in this book are meant to inspire the reader to learn from the process of failures to achieve success. In retrospect, the failures appear obvious, but all attempts to innovate require innovative thinking, and the reader is encouraged to read each story keeping in mind the facts known at the time the work was being conducted.

Summation:

This book has also been inspired by several scientists who have authored the stories of their personal experiences. The most difficult skill of a scientist is the ability to communicate the complexities of discoveries and inventions to the lay person. I have used anecdotes, real-life stories and conversations with the people involved in the stories to narrate the development of novel drugs for the treatment of difficult diseases. The common thread that weaves through this book is the inflection point. Each story has one. It was not obvious at the start of the experience, nor even midway, but it was realized retrospectively after success was observed. This book is part of my experiment with a process of self-awareness. I have written extensively about this process, which I urge the reader to follow on my blog (chirmule.wordpress.com).

Readers are also encouraged to watch my TEDx talk on YouTube.[*]

This book also focuses on delineating the mechanisms of failure and understanding the processes of learning and other factors that may lead to success. Several articles have studied the concepts of failure.[†] These studies have been done in the areas of scientific grants, start-ups and terrorism. Chance and learning are the mechanisms of recovering from failures in these diverse areas. The number of attempts to recover is exponentially related to the probability of success. A major point gleaned from these studies is that valuable lessons are difficult to learn without experiencing failure. Detecting the signs of potential failure will allow a deeper understanding of the complex dynamics involved in achieving success.

The failures articulated in the seven stories of drug development in biotechnology in this book are all followed by success. The lessons learnt during the process have enabled the listing of many aspects that can be applied

---

[*] Chirmule, N. TEDx Presentation. 'Biotechnology'. https://www.youtube.com/watch?v=IXilhg-34SQ).

[†] 1. Yin, Y., Wang, Y., Evans, J.A. and Wang, D. 'Quantifying the Dynamics of Failure across Science, Startups and Security'. *Nature* 575 (2019): 190–94.

2. Sitkin, S.B. 'Learning through Failure. The Strategy of Small Losses'. *Research in Organizational Behaviours*. 14 (1992) 231–66.

3. Fortunato, S., Bergstrom, C.T., Börner, K., Evans, J.A., Helbing, D., Milojevi,S.,Petersen,A.M.,Radicchi,F.,Sinatra,R.,Uzzi,B.,Vespignani,A., Waltman, L., Wang, D. and Barabási, A.L. 'Science of Science'. *Science* 359 (2018) 1–7. DOI: 10.1126/science.aao0185.

to life stories. Making your own journey of successes and failures will enable you to find inflection points that changed your course. Finding these inflection points is an interesting exercise in self-awareness and can be used repeatedly on the path to progress.

1

The Story of Haemophilia

Murali's courageous journey in haemophilia—which he
considers 'his normal life'.

The year was 1986. We were young, twenty-four-year-
old PhD students of immunology at the prestigious
Cancer Research Institute at Mumbai's Tata Hospital, an
institution dedicated to research into understanding the
mechanism of cancer. We were conducting experiments
with patient samples and just starting to learn the process
of conducting research. We were attempting to decipher
why cancer cells in patients grew uncontrollably and
what biological systems were required to keep the cell
growth in control. It was our first exposure to basic
research and discovery. We were enthusiastic and full of
young energy, having just graduated and been given the
amazing opportunity to work with the best in the field of
cancer biology. Murali Pazhayannur was a fellow student

and one of my best friends. We were in the immunology programme, led by Sudha Gangal, and were working on aspects of basic immunology, such as T cell and B cell functions. It was a time when the functions of these cells were being discovered. The immunology textbooks had not yet been written. The work was intense, and one activity of camaraderie that we did together as students was to go hiking. We were planning a trip to Igatpuri, a hill station near Mumbai, and were high on enthusiasm about things to take and things to do. Murali was as enthusiastic as we were, maybe more. One thing we knew, but did not appreciate the gravitas of back then, was that Murali had haemophilia—a genetic disease that causes severe bleeding. During the trip, unbeknownst to us, Murali had had several episodes of internal and external bleeding, each one of which could have been traumatic. However, the process of dealing with these bleeds, that he had developed to deal with the life-threatening problems, were 'just taken care of', and we never knew about them. Only years later did Murali and I talk about these everyday episodes of bleeding that are part of his life. A lesson for all of us from this episode, is the 'deal with our problems and use the solutions we have without making a fuss'.[*]

The process of clotting of blood involves a series of sequential proteins that culminate in a blood clot, which is

---

[*] Murali, P.S.M. 'Choices you make, the chances you take'. https://www.youtube.com/watch?v=Ohe5Gtn56Dk&t=82s

a mesh of proteins. Haemophilia is caused by a mutation in a gene that encodes a protein. Thirteen proteins, called factors and numbered as factor I to XIII, are involved in the clotting process. Each factor in the cascade is an enzyme that is not active unless activated by the previous one. Finally, these proteins activate the mesh-forming proteins thrombin and fibrin, which form the blood clot within minutes of a wound being inflicted. In the normal course, the complex clotting process occurs so seamlessly and predictably that we do not pay attention to the mechanisms involved from cut to clot. The proteins involved in the clotting process sequentially activate the next in a cascade, like the game passing-the-parcel. When the music stops (i.e., when there is a mutation in a protein in that sequence), the blood fails to clot. Since the blood does not clot, wounds do not heal, and as a result patients can die of excessive bleeding. Patients have different levels of deficiency from severe (less than 1 per cent of the normal factor levels), to moderate (1 to 5 per cent of the normal factor levels) to mild (5 to 40 per cent of the normal factor levels).

Murali has a mutation in the factor VIII protein. When he has an injury, his blood fails to clot. He would have internal bleeding even after climbing a flight of stairs (as he told us later).

So how did Murali survive given that his blood does not clot?

In 1965, Murali, then a normal five-year-old boy in Calcutta, underwent a routine procedure of having his tonsils removed due to a persistent bacterial infection. During the surgery, he kept bleeding as his blood failed to clot. He was diagnosed with haemophilia by an American doctor working at Christian Medical College in Vellore. He was treated with a transfusion of fresh whole blood from an ABO blood-type matched healthy donor. He was then given transfusions once or twice a year for the next ten years, until he was eighteen years old. The only treatment available was encapsulated in an acronym: RICE, or rest, icing, compression and elevation.

In 1979, Murali suffered a hip injury when he fell off a hand-pulled rickshaw in Calcutta. He lost a lot of blood. Murali's parents were in Bombay, and he was living with a close school friend, Hemant Mehta, and his parents. He was hospitalized. A young doctor at the hospital knew of a product called cryoprecipitate to treat haemophilia. There was a frantic search for this cryoprecipitate. His father contacted everyone he knew and was able to obtain the product, which was procured from Haffkine Institute in Bombay and then shipped to Calcutta in dry ice, on a commercial flight. Murali survived. Fortunate patients like Murali who had access to the life-saving treatments of cryoprecipitate or plasma transfusions could be treated whenever they encountered bleeds. But for millions of patients with haemophilia, there were no options.

Murali finished high school after taking a break in class eleven to recover from the bleed caused by the hip fracture. He then went on to do his bachelor's and master's degrees in microbiology from Bhavan's College at the University of Bombay. In October 1985, he joined the PhD programme at the Cancer Research Institute, in Parel, Bombay. This was a remarkable achievement for a boy with such a severe bleeding disorder. Every activity he undertook required careful planning and execution. But the disease did not diminish the enthusiasm and ambition of this young man.

Murali has always been extremely talkative. During our college years, he would tell us endless stories in his flamboyantly enthusiastic style. In a contemporary play loosely based on the Ramayana that we had acted in, he played King Dasharatha. He has always been the king of his thoughts, always focused on his goals in life. Never did we consider him to be suffering from a disease that could take his life at any moment.

Haemophilia is a death sentence to about one in 15,000 births. That frequency works out to about 1,50,000 children in India. The official registry of haemophilia patients in India lists approximately 30,000 patients. Murali has the most severe form of the disease. His cells do not have the gene for factor VIII and thus they do not make any clotting factor. Yet, through the miracles of his support system, his family, friends and doctors, he has not just survived, but made enormous contributions to society, especially to the community of those suffering from haemophilia in India and the US.

Treatments for haemophilia[*]

Cryoprecipitate

From the 1920s to the 1950s, RICE and fresh whole blood transfusions were the only treatments available for those suffering from haemophilia. In 1965, Dr Judith Graham Pool, a professor of medicine at the Stanford University School of Medicine, discovered a frozen precipitate from plasma, called cryoprecipitate.[†] It was obtained through a process that enabled serum clotting factors to be precipitated in very cold conditions, which could then be stored and later transfused into patients. This cryoprecipitate contained the suite of proteins involved in the clotting cascade (such as factors VII, VIII, IX, the von Willebrand factor, etc.) purified from the blood of healthy individuals. This process was widely used and radically improved the access to life-saving clotting factors for patients all around the world.

Blood transfusions or administering cryoprecipitate from healthy volunteers was an effective therapy for managing the disease. Then, in the early 1980s, disaster struck. Blood banks in the US as well as India were contaminated with the AIDS virus. Transfusions of this contaminated blood wreaked havoc by infecting thousands

---

[*] Hemophilia: From Plasma to Recombinant Factors. https://www.hematology.org/about/history/50-years/hemophilia (accessed on 14 May 2021).

[†] Kasper, C.K. 'Judith Graham Pool and the Discovery of Cryoprecipitate'. *Hemophilia* 18 (2012): 833–35.

of haemophiliacs. This was a huge price paid by the haemophiliac community (patients and their families) due to the oversight by the blood collection centres and regulators. Only a miracle saved Murali. He had completed his PhD and moved to the Medical College of Wisconsin in Milwaukee in the US for his post-doctoral research. By this time the US Food and Drug Administration (FDA) had created a quality approval system in the blood banks in the US to ensure screening of blood for HIV.

However, there was a great unmet need to provide an alternative solution to the blood-derived clotting factors.

Recombinant factors

It was the beginning of the biotechnology revolution in San Francisco. The scientists at the American biotechnology company Genentech had sequenced the gene that encoded factor VIII and shared the results in a publication in *Nature* magazine in 1984.* An innovative treatment from the field of biotechnology came from a technique called recombinant DNA in molecular biology. The process of recombination is a mixing of gene segments, whereby genes on a chromosome can be cut and placed in a different order. This process, which occurs naturally,

---

* Gitschier, J., Wood, W.I., Goralka, T.M., Wion, K.L., Chen, E.Y., Eaton, D.H., Vehar, G., Capon, D.J. and Lawn, D.J. 'Characterization of the Human Factor VIII Gene'. *Nature* 312 (1984): 330–7.

for example, when virus genes enter the host genome, was exploited by researchers at Baxter, a company that had been purifying the haemophilia factors from blood for many years. They developed a method to make the clotting factors by inserting the genes for the factors into the genome of bacteria (*Escerechia Coli*). These bacteria, which were genetically transformed by the insertion of the human factor VIII gene, secreted this clotting factor, which was purified from the bacterial material into a clear solution (buffer). The factor VIII protein solution was then carefully placed in vials so it could be drawn out through a syringe and administered into the vein of a patient to control bleeding. The intravenous injection. The treatment of haemophiliacs no longer required blood transfusions, which eliminated the risk of being infected with HIV and other blood-borne viruses. This was a remarkable step forward in the treatment of haemophilia. The commercial product was called Recombinate®, which was approved by the FDA in 1992. Similarly, the other clotting factors were also made by recombinant technology. The treatment of haemophiliacs with recombinant clotting factors has provided convenience and safety against blood-borne infections like HIV.

In order to manage his bleeding, Murali takes an intravenous injection of recombinant factor VIII every other day. It is quite a laborious and intense process. He arranges all the materials on a clean sheet of paper spread out on his dining table at home. He then warms the region of his hand or arm where he will self-administer the injection. He combines the two sections of the vial containing the recombinant factor VIII by shaking it thoroughly to mix the ingredients in the two compartments (one a concentrate of factor VIII protein powder, and the other the diluent). The device, which includes the drug (factor VIII protein), the water (to dissolve the drug) and filter, that Murali uses to inject himself with the factor VIII, enables the mixing of the solutions before injection. He rests after the injection.

This single injection costs $4500. He must take it every other day. The average cost per year is a staggering $81,900 for prophylaxis and more if he has bleeding events, for which he requires the injection twice a day. Murali's insurance company pays for the treatment. He is fortunate to work for a company that provides this coverage.

In India, the availability of the clotting factors is extremely low. Not only is the amount of clotting factors that need to be injected to maintain a minimal level of these factors much lower, but the cost is approximately Rs 20,000 ($275). Due to the lack of regular availability of the factor in hospitals and pharmacies, especially in rural areas, it is given only sparingly to patients who require it the most, during bleeding episodes. The challenge of managing the disease has economic, personal, familial, social, emotional and psychological layers. The patient along with the caregiver may have to miss several days of work or school. In addition, there is significant pain, both physical and mental. *Will innovation in* *biotechnology come to the rescue?* Indian pharmaceutical companies still do not make the recombinant protein. It requires a significant investment of millions of dollars in infrastructure, understanding the science and technology behind the production, and patent protection. Further, the financial return on investment is low, since there are a relatively small number of haemophiliacs in the country.* *So how does a company get its returns?* The answers to these questions are still being addressed.

Hemlibra®†

A major challenge in the treatment of haemophilia is the formation of inhibitors (neutralizing antibodies). For patients with the clotting factor mutation, the normal form of the protein will be foreign to the immune system. Hence many patients develop antibodies against the haemophilia factors. This event is lethal to patients, in that replacement therapy with the factors is made non-functional by the antibodies.

On one spectacular day in March 2015, as we sat in a beautiful café in Santa Monica, Murali was explaining the mechanism of a novel drug for the treatment of a subset of haemophiliacs being developed by Genentech. The treatment is called Hemlibra®. It utilizes the unique ability

---

* Hemophilia Federation of India (HFI). https://www.hemophilia.in/
† Hemlibra Prescribing Information. https://www.hemlibra.com/ (accessed on 14 May 2021)

of antibody molecules to bind to two separate clotting factors. The structure of an antibody looks something like the letter Y. One tip of the Y of the antibody molecule binds to factor VII and the other tip binds to factor IX, thereby bridging the clotting cascade without the requirement of factor VIII. This novel invention was an outcome of the work done on developing antibodies as drugs. This drug is lifesaving for haemophiliacs who develop inhibitors to factor VIII. It took many years to develop this molecule and make it available for patients. Murali was part of the patient advisory board for Genentech's scientific group.

A few years later in May 2019, I watched Murali as he sat at his dining table and injected himself with Hemlibra®. The use of Hemlibra® has significantly lowered the number of factor infusions he needs in case of a major bleed. The value of developing drugs becomes real to a scientist of the trade only when the impact is seen on the patient's life. Watching Murali take this drug, which had a major impact on his quality of life (since he now had to take injections less frequently), was one such moment for me, as I have spent the better part of my life working on the development of drugs. It is all about the patient, ultimately.

Gene therapy for haemophilia

The recombinant factor, while an effective treatment, is not a cure for the disease. The holy grail of the treatment of genetic diseases is gene therapy. The normal gene that encodes for the clotting factor can be inserted into the cell of a person suffering from haemophilia, which in turn can cure the disease.

The story of gene therapy started many years ago and was conceptualized when the techniques to manipulate genes and put them into a cell were developed and perfected.

Let us first understand what a gene is. A gene is a unit of hereditary information that can be transmitted to your children. It is transmitted as a whole unit, carries specific information, and determines the appearance, fate and future of your children. It is made up of a chemical substance called nucleotide. There are four nucleotides: A, C, T and G. These nucleotides, in various permutations and combinations, spell out our entire genome. A mutation in any of these nucleotides causes some dysfunction of the gene and results in a disease.

On 14 September 1990, Ashanti DeSilva was the first patient to be treated with gene therapy under the direction of William French Anderson and Michael Blaese at the National Institutes of Health (NIH) in Bethesda.[*] The disease was an immune disorder caused by a mutation of a gene for the enzyme adenosine deaminase (ADA) in the cells of the bone marrow. The cells of the bone marrow are stem cells for the cells of the immune system. Due to this mutation the bone marrow cells of a person suffering from this disease have severe (combined) immune

---

[*] Naam, R. 'More than Human'. *New York Times*, 3 July 2005.

deficiency (SCID). Without the immune system, the patient is susceptible to bacterial and viral infections.

Drs Anderson and Blaese developed a virus that contained the normal ADA gene, infected Ashanti's bone marrow cells with it and transplanted them back. Astonishingly, the treatment was a success.* Her immune system developed completely. She went back to school and today, she is a young woman pursuing a normal life. The success of this trial marked the beginning of the field of gene therapy. But not all trials had such success stories.

In Murali's case, he has a mutation in a few nucleotides in a gene that encodes for the protein factor VIII, the absence of which prevents blood from clotting. Giving the normal gene to Murali should be able to correct his disease. But it is not that easy. Before we come back to treating Murali's haemophilia by gene therapy, we need to understand why it is so difficult. We have to encounter the story of another genetic disease, of courage, tragedy and perseverance. (See Jim Wilson's story on the development of viral vectors for gene therapy in Chapter 6.)

The positive attitude towards life that Murali had when we were in college continues to this day. He now lives in Chicago, where he works as a database administrator for a financial institution. He is happily married, and he and his wife Sridevi have a son. The difficulties Murali must undergo just to survive would shame any one of us when

---

* Naam, R. 'More than Human'. *New York Times*, 3 July 2005.

we complain of the smallest paper cut. He has taught me so many lessons in living every moment of life to the fullest. In April 2019, he was awarded the Volunteer of the Year by the Hemophilia Federation of America.

2

The Rotavirus Vaccine

The story of preventing diarrhoea and death in children:
the dichotomy of the developed and underdeveloped worlds.

Vaccines are one of mankind's greatest innovations in biotechnology and have saved millions of lives by protecting us against infectious diseases. Today, every child on earth can be vaccinated with a series of vaccines that prevent death at an early age. Before vaccines, infant mortality due to infections was extremely common. Vaccines against the measles, mumps, rubella and varicella (chicken pox) viruses, as well as against diphtheria, tetanus and pertussis among others, are now routinely given to children.

The story of the measles vaccine

Measles is a highly contagious viral infection that is transmitted by airborne droplets. The infection results in a severe rash throughout the body, a telltale sign of the disease. Seven to eight million children died every year of the measles infection until the vaccine was developed in 1963; the number is now down to a few hundred.* We take protection against measles for granted. The World Health Organization (WHO) has declared it to be next in line to be eradicated from the world, after smallpox and polio.† It is rare to see a patient with measles, let alone die of it. It was not so in the past.

The story of vaccines started with an experiment done by Nature and observed by humans. Peter Panum, a Danish physiologist and pathologist, was sent by the government to study a measles outbreak in the Faroe Islands of Denmark, which lie between Iceland and Scotland (Panum, 1846).‡ Panum wrote in great detail about his five-month sojourn on the islands, where people kept their stoves burning in the cold summer temperatures. His paper, which is considered a medical classic, states that 'people developed the measles rash approximately fourteen days after exposure to the infective matter, and that surviving the infection resulted in lifelong immunity against the disease.'

Humans, and yes only humans not animals, get infected in the lungs with the measles virus by breathing. It is one

---

* Measles (Ruboela). Centers for Disease Control. https://www.cdc.gov/measles/index.html
† 'Eliminating Measles and Rubella: Framework for the Verification Process in the WHO European Region'. (2014).
‡ Panum, P. 'Observations Made during the Epidemic of Measles during the Year 1846'. *Medical Classic* 3 (1939): 879–86.

of the most transmittable diseases, several times more so than HIV and Ebola. It enters the lining of the lung, starts dividing and then spreads to the lymph nodes. If the virus manages to get to the brain, it causes severe permanent damage to the nervous system. A battle between the virus and immune system ensues. For most healthy people, the immune system wins. For about 10 to 25 per cent of the population (depending on age, region and other factors), the virus is lethal. The immune system is not able to contain it and patients die of secondary infections such as pneumonia. It takes about fourteen days for the virus to be cleared by the immune system. This fact was noted by Peter Panum in 1846 when neither was the virus known nor was it understood that the immune system was responsible for its clearance. The patient at this stage of the infection is highly contagious. The virus enters the respiratory system through the nose. Sick patients transmit the virus through nasal secretions or sneezing, where each droplet contains thousands of virus particles. And so the disease spreads. Each patient can infect about seven to fourteen individuals. Relatively, a patient suffering from the Ebola virus (which caused outbreaks in 1976, 2014–16, 2018–20 and most recently from 7 February–3 May 2021)* can infect only two individuals.

Back to the story in the Faroe Islands in the summer of 1846. Peter Panum noticed that while measles was a childhood disease, it attacked the entire population of the

---

* https://www.who.int/emergencies/situations/ebola-2021-north-kivu

island. He wrote in his historic paper about the daughter of a farmer named J. Hansen, who was also a churchwarden. She infected nine other members of the household. Because of his keen observations, Peter Panum deduced that once one person in a household was infected, others would follow suit. The most interesting fact that emerged from his important medical observations was that despite the virulence, inhabitants of the Faroe Islands who had had the measles sixty-five years earlier escaped infection. This report was the first that suggested the possibility of prevention of infections by vaccinations, even before it was known how measles was transmitted. In fact, it would take approximately another hundred years for the measles virus to be discovered.

Thomas C. Peebles (1921–2010), along with John Franklin Enders, isolated the virus from an eleven-year-old boy, David Edmonston, in Boston, in 1954. Enders, who won the Nobel Prize in Physiology or Medicine in 1954 for isolating the polio virus, is considered the father of modern vaccines.[*]

In another part of the world, the American microbiologist Maurice Hilleman and his colleagues at Merck in West Point, Philadelphia, developed the vaccine to prevent measles in 1963 from a measles virus isolated from his daughter, Jeryl-Lynn. Both Edmonston and Jeryl-Lynn

---

[*] Griffin D., Oldstone, M.B.A. 'Measles. History and Basic Biology', *Curr. Top, Microbiol. Immunol.* (2009), 329:1.

are names of strains of measles viruses. The principle of the vaccine was to give a 'non-infectious virus' as a vaccine, which would in turn activate the immune system to make antibodies, which in turn would block the measles virus from infecting the lungs. We take this mechanism of action of the vaccine for granted. Maurice Hilleman and many of his peers developed several vaccines, such as those against rubella and mumps, which have prevented millions of deaths.

But the development of vaccines is not a financially lucrative business. The cost of development is in the hundreds of millions of dollars. Also, there is a very high requirement of efficacy and safety. Thus, the unrealistic expectations of a vaccine are that it should be 100 per cent efficacious (i.e., the vaccine should work for everyone), there should be no side effects and it should be free. An impossible task in drug development. Despite these massive challenges, there is a desperate need to vaccinate billions of people against a variety of diseases so that they do not die.

We must therefore ask, why is it so expensive to develop a vaccine? Why are the expectations of a vaccine so high? Let us look at the story of the vaccine against rotavirus infection as an example.

The story of the rotavirus vaccine

It was a turning point in the history of vaccines. The day was 10 October 2010. The place, the Supreme Court of the United States, and the case, Bruesewitz versus Wyeth LLC.

The pharmaceutical company Wyeth LLC was being held accountable for the death and severe adverse events caused by the administration of the rotavirus vaccine to twenty-eight children. The case presented evidence for and against the cause of death by the vaccine to be associated with a rare intestinal condition, called intussusception, which is a telescoping of the intestine, resulting in blockage. In February 2011, the court ruled in favour of Wyeth LLC, and in doing so limiting the liability of civil claims. The case was seen as a victory for vaccine manufacturing companies. As is the case in many landmark verdicts, the case was neither a resounding loss nor victory for society at large.

Until recently, more than five hundred thousand children in the world died of diarrhoeal diseases every year. There are many organisms that infect the gut and cause severe disease, especially in children. Salmonella and E. coli are the most common. Among viruses, one of the most virulent is rotavirus. It is highly contagious and causes severe disease, including diarrhoea, which results in dehydration and ultimately death. Most children in the US and European countries who are infected with rotavirus and are seriously ill are hospitalized and treated. In countries where the healthcare system is poor, many children die. Until 1998 there was no vaccine to prevent rotavirus infection.

Wyeth (now a wholly owned subsidiary of Pfizer Inc.) undertook the Herculean task of developing a vaccine against rotavirus in the 1980s. Generally, the steps for developing a vaccine are as follows:

1. Design a strain of the virus that does not replicate in humans
2. Develop a process to manufacture this attenuated (weakened) strain
3. Utilize analytics to determine the attributes of the vaccine that impart its efficacy
4. Test it for safety in animals
5. Test it in normal healthy humans for side effects
6. Test it in humans to ensure it protects against infections and disease by comparing with a control (placebo) group of subjects
7. Obtain approval from the regulatory agencies

Wyeth submitted the data package for approval in 1996. The process from design to approval took fifteen years and cost hundreds of millions of dollars.*

The Wyeth vaccine was developed by virologist Albert Kapikian and his colleagues at the National Institutes of Health in Bethesda who designed the vaccine by utilizing the property of a strain of rotavirus found in rhesus monkeys. This strain is markedly less virulent in humans. The proteins on the virus that are responsible for activating the human immune system to develop a protective response were determined by extensive experiments in mice and rats. These proteins (VP4, VP6)

---

* Rennels, M.B. 'The Rotavirus Vaccine Story: A Clinical Investigator's View'. *Pediatrics* (2000): 1–10.

are expressed on the surface of the virus. Their function is to bind to specific molecules to enter human cells. Antibodies generated by the immune systems of humans bind to these viral proteins and prevent the virus from entering the epithelial cells of the gut, thereby preventing rotavirus infection-induced pathological effects. These types of antibodies are named neutralizing antibodies. Therefore, the vaccine was designed by combining the beneficial properties of the protection-inducing components of the human rotavirus (VP4, VP6) and the attenuated replicative components of the rhesus rotavirus. The process of combining viruses is called reassortment. The virulence property of the vaccine product is required to enable the virus to grow in cells, so that the vaccine can be manufactured inside cells. The vaccine is made by infecting cells growing in large bioreactors with live virus (reassorted to contain the envelope proteins of the human rotavirus, packaged in a rhesus monkey rotavirus). To add to the complexity of the vaccine, there are several strains of rotavirus that are prevalent in humans. The vaccine should be capable of protecting against all the major strains. Thus, the reassorted vaccine, which was made of four different strains of the human rotavirus (tetravalent vaccine), was tested in preclinical studies to demonstrate safety and evaluate the side effects. Twenty-seven clinical trials covering 10,000 children in nine countries, primarily in South America and Europe, were conducted. The criterion for the double-blind clinical trial was to assess the ability of the vaccine to protect more than 80 per cent of the vaccinated children from rotavirus infection.

The evaluation of the safety and efficacy of the vaccine was done by the FDA, along with the Vaccines and Related Biological Products Advisory Committee (VRBPAC), and the Rotavirus Working Group of the Advisory Committee on Immunization Practices (ACIP) of the Centers for Disease Control and Prevention (CDC), a common practice. This group comprises experts from different areas, including paediatric infectious disease, vaccine immunology and manufacturing, epidemiology and policymakers in public health. The results of the vaccine development process, including all the toxicology reports, manufacturing processes and clinical trials, were presented and discussed in a six-hour meeting in December 1997. The vaccine demonstrated a 69 to 91 per cent efficacy in protecting against diarrhoea, depending on the strain of rotavirus. This level of protection was similar to that of other vaccines.

During the course of the review process, Dr Carolyn Hardegree, director of the Office of Vaccine Research and Review at the FDA, and other members noted that one of the safety events observed was intussusception. Intussusception is a prolapsing of a part of the intestine into another section of the intestine, similar to a collapsible telescope. This condition is a medical emergency that causes obstruction of the gut, loss of oxygen to the intestine resulting in gangrene, intestinal perforation and ultimately death. Treatment is surgical intervention. Dr Margaret Rennels, a professor at the University of Maryland, led the multicentre clinical trial and reported on behalf of Wyeth. Out of the 10,054 vaccinated children, five had reported intussusception, three of which occurred during the first week after receiving the vaccine, and one child among 4633 placebo recipients also developed the condition. During the course of a trial, the clinical trial investigators (doctors) are responsible for managing the vaccine recipients and reporting any adverse event that occurs due to the vaccine. In this case, none of the cases of intussusception were judged by the investigators to be associated with the vaccine. The five vaccinated individuals who had experienced intussusception had participated in five different clinical trials and had received three different rhesus rotavirus vaccine preparations, each with a different manufacturing process. It was concluded that the association of intussusception with the vaccinated individuals was due to temporal chance, since the rate of this rare condition observed in the clinical trial was not different to that observed in the general population and reported in the literature. After a detailed review of the safety and efficacy of the clinical data, it was determined that the vaccine provided greater benefit than risk and was approved for use on 31 August 1998. It was named RotaShield®. American Home Products (AHP), the parent company of Wyeth, touted the vaccine as a 'breakthrough therapy for a severe disease'.

The excitement over the availability of a vaccine to prevent diarrhoea and associated hospitalization of children in the US resulted in high sales. Priced at $116 for the three doses, it was a high revenue generator for the company. About a million children were dosed.

A year later, the vaccine was removed from the market. What happened?

In the US, while the FDA is responsible for review and approval of vaccines, another government agency oversees the use of the vaccine: CDC. It does so through the ACIP. This committee had also reviewed the data from the clinical trials for the vaccine and had approved the recommendation to vaccinate all children with three doses of RotaShield® at two, four and six months from birth.

The Vaccine Adverse Reporting System (VARES) of the CDC was established as a reporting mechanism for doctors, patients or anyone else observing any side effects of vaccines. The process is known as pharmacovigilance. It is a process of self-reporting through which the CDC reviews and determines the continued efficacy and safety of any product that is approved. In 1999, sixty-two cases of adverse events related to RotaShield® were reported, of which three were intussusception. More cases began to be reported. The ACIP met in June 1999 to review these reports. Following the review, the committee recommended temporarily suspending the vaccine until further review. The news of the potential severe side effects of the rotavirus vaccine hit the front page of the *New York Times*. Eighty-three more cases were reported to the VARES in July. Several investigations were undertaken to determine the association of the vaccine with the rare condition. The most conclusive study compared 429 children with intussusception between November 1998 and June 1999, to 1763 non-vaccinated children. The results showed that RotaShield®-vaccinated children had a statistically higher probability of developing the intestinal blockade syndrome. The ACIP meeting to discuss the data from these cases was scheduled for October 1999. A week before the meeting, anticipating its outcome, Wyeth recalled the vaccine from the market on 15 October 1999.*

The government stated: '. . . events surrounding the withdrawal of the RotaShield® vaccine illustrate how well this system functions in practice.' In the space of about one year, a vaccine was licensed and recommended for routine administration, adverse events raised a concern, further studies were conducted, and the manufacturer withdrew the vaccine knowing the government and physician community were ready to respond.†

The withdrawal of RotaShield® from the market was a major setback for the millions of children who were dying from rotavirus infections every day. In the US, in 1998,

* Altman, L. 'Vaccine for Infant Diarrhea is Withdrawn as Health Risk', *New York Times*, 16 October 1999.
† Schwartz, J. 'The First Rotavirus Vaccine and Politics of Acceptable Risk', *Millbank Q*. 2012 Jun; 90 (2): 278–310.

before the vaccine was available, approximately three million children had rotavirus infection-induced stomach upsets, which required more than 6,00,000 doctor visits and around 70,000 hospitalizations, which added to the burden of cost to the healthcare system. However, due to the access to simple rehydration therapies in the US, the number of deaths was less than 100 per year. The story worldwide, however, was very different. More than 5,00,000 children died of rotavirus infections every year. The social considerations of the diametrically different outcomes of the rotavirus infections led to discussions on ethical considerations to determine whether RotaShield® could benefit children worldwide, despite the risk. The discussion was sealed shut after a meeting of experts from the fields of medicine and ethics, social workers and government agencies in 2000 at the WHO offices in Geneva. As one minister put it, 'If the vaccine is not good enough for the children in the US, it is not good for theirs either.'*

The disastrous experience with the RotaShield® vaccine was not the first of its kind. Serious adverse events after vaccinations had occurred in the past. The polio vaccine, developed by American virologist and medical researcher Jonas Salk and his colleagues in 1955 and manufactured by Cutter Laboratories, resulted in thousands of children

---

* Schwartz, J. 'The First Rotavirus Vaccine and Politics of Acceptable Risks'. *Millbank Q*. 2012 Jun; 90 (2): 278–310.

being exposed to a live polio virus, leading to ten deaths and many more children getting paralysis. In 1976, a high incidence of Guillain-Barre Syndrome—a rare disorder in which the body's immune system attacks the nerves, eventually paralysing the whole body—was observed in the military when the swine flu virus vaccine was administered. The vaccination was halted. Since then, several lawsuits have been filed regarding the potential association of vaccinations with various conditions. The most notorious being the association of autism with vaccines, which was published by the former physician and academic Andrew Wakefield. His paper has been retracted for falsifying data, but not before it caused a huge outcry and spawned numerous conspiracy theories.

There was thus an urgent and desperate need for a vaccine to prevent rotavirus infection. In this climate and under these circumstances, nothing short of courage was required to propose another live virus vaccine to prevent rotavirus infections. It was around this time, in 1998, that Professors Fred Clark and Paul Offit from the University of Pennsylvania (UPenn), and Roger Glass a scientist at the CDC were working on alternative vaccinations against the rotavirus. The team was collaborating with the pharma company Merck in Philadelphia to develop a vaccine. I was at Merck at that time (from 2000 to 2007). I led the bioanalytical team and worked very closely with Fred Clark and the students and post-doctoral fellows in his lab at Children's Hospital of Philadelphia (CHOP).

Dan DiStefano, a stocky, extremely diligent scientist, led the molecular biology team at Merck. His team was instrumental in developing all the virus detection methods. No small task since the virus was shed and had to be detected from the diapers of babies with rotavirus infection. James Drummond, a calm and extremely thoughtful scientist at Merck, led the team that was responsible for measuring immune responses to the vaccine. The statistical team was led by Joseph Heyes, and the clinical team by Penny Heaton, both at Merck.* Penny later became the CEO of the Bill and Melinda Gates Foundation. Jacqueline Miller, a nephrologist, had just completed her fellowship at CHOP, and joined the Merck clinical team at the suggestion of Paul Offit. Jackie is now the head of the clinical team at Moderna, which developed one of the mRNA vaccines against COVID-19.

When the news of intussusceptions emerged from studies of RotaShield®, there was a high degree of nervousness in the Children's Hospital of Philadelphia (CHOP)-Merck camp. Millions of dollars were being invested to conduct large clinical trials to demonstrate the efficacy and safety of the vaccine. Not only would it be a financial disaster to proceed, but the vaccine could also cause harm to children

---

* Heyes, J., Kuter, B., Dallas, M.J. and Heaton, P. 'Evaluating the Safety of the Rotavirus Vaccines; the REST of the Study'. Clinical Trials 5 (2008): 131–9.

in the trial. A major decision had to be made. Should we proceed with the development of the rotavirus vaccine?

The team was busy calculating the size of the trial that would be required to confirm that the vaccine would not cause intussusception. This uncommon condition has an incidence of eighteen to fifty-six cases per 1,00,000 infants during the first year of life in the US. The population attributable risk (PAR)—the proportion of the incidence of a disease in the population (exposed and unexposed) that is due to exposure—detected in the post-marketing studies for RotaShield® was approximately one case per 10,000 vaccine recipients. The Merck rotavirus vaccine clinical trial was in the midst of Phase II, and the decision to proceed to Phase III required data to understand two major risks: the safety of the vaccine, and the potential loss of millions of dollars if the vaccine study failed.

The Merck vaccine, called RotaTeq®, comprised the surface proteins of four strains of the human rotavirus (tetravalent) combined with the bovine rotavirus backbone (i.e. the combination of the bovine and human rotaviruses that render the vaccine non-infectious). The initial data from clinical efficacy trails was highly encouraging with 70–100 per cent of the vaccinated children being protected from diarrhoeal episodes. No cases of intussusception had been observed in the studies thus far. Epidemiological studies had suggested that there was no association of intussusception with the human rotavirus infection. Animal studies by Merck had also shown some differences from the

Wyeth vaccine. Based on this data, Merck's management made the decision to proceed with Phase III of the clinical trial. Due to the potential risk of intussusception, it was critical to evaluate the safety of the vaccine with a very large clinical trial. Indeed, it was the largest Phase III clinical trial ever done.

The Rotavirus Efficacy and Safety Trial (REST) was a double-blind study conducted in eleven countries at over 500 study sites.* Half the children received the vaccine, and half the placebo. The study involved approximately 70,000 subjects. As the study was double-blind, neither the subjects nor the doctors administering the vaccine (or placebo) knew what they were receiving or giving. This meticulous process was required to avoid bias in the results. Such clinical studies are monitored by an unblinded Data Safety Monitoring Board (DSMB), which comprises doctors, statisticians and clinical study management scientists, who are experts in the field, but not part of the study team.

The design of the REST study had three major challenges. It had to: i) include a large enough number of subjects so as to determine the risk of a rare side effect; ii) monitor the occurrence of intussusception in tens of thousands of children; and iii) ensure the study was conducted under the

---

* Heyes, J., Kuter, B., Dallas, M.J. and Heaton, P. 'Evaluating the Safety of the Rotavirus Vaccines; the REST of the Study'. Clinical Trials 5 (2008): 131–9.

regulatory processes so that the data could demonstrate the efficacy and safety of the vaccine.

Earlier studies had suggested that three shots of the vaccine given within six months of age were required for an effective immune response to be generated by the child. The immune response was measured forty-two days after each dose. It is known that the peak age at which rotavirus infection occurs is between six and twenty-four months. This is also the age range when the background rates of intussusception increase, i.e., the rates of intussusception of children in the general population. If the number of cases of intussusception increased in the study, it would provide a signal to stop the study early. The study team developed a detailed plan to administer the vaccine and placebo and determine efficacy by documenting cases of diarrhoea, and safety by monitoring the incidence of intussusception.

Thus, the clinical study defined its end points for safety as follows: i) through continuous monitoring of the vaccine and placebo subjects, determine that the number of intussusception cases is below the prespecified numbers during the course of the study, based on the incidence of one in 1,00,000 cases; and ii) at the end of the study, the group receiving the vaccine does not have a higher risk of intussusception than the placebo group.

To appreciate the gravitas of this study design, consider the following points. Each increment of 10,000 subjects in a clinical trial can cost the company at least $100 million;

and with a rare occurrence there should be only ten cases of intussusception with 1,00,000 children administered either the vaccine or the placebo. We should note that the probability of intussusception occurring in either vaccine or placebo group should be equal, or else the study would be void. The stakes were very high. The statisticians designed a graph that showed a boundary comparing vaccine and placebo treated subjects. If any case that was reported fell into the 'grey zone', the study would fail. Remember, it was a double-blind study, and only the DSMB knew the result. In the field of drug development, this study was akin to 'sitting on the edge of your seat'.

Before undertaking such a high-risk project, the statisticians conducted a simulation experiment to calculate the probability of a successful outcome. A computer program randomly determined 10,000 subjects to be given three doses of vaccine or placebo, followed by randomly assigning intussusception to one in every 10,000 subjects. For each case, the computer program determined whether the increasing number of cases of intussusception fell between the boundaries of the predefined expected values in the graph (grey zone). The software calculated a 0.06 per cent risk that the study would need to be stopped early due to a safety event, and a 94 per cent probability that the study would reach a successful outcome if approximately 1,00,000 children were enrolled in the study. The simulation also calculated the relative risks in real-time when subjects were being enrolled, since the smaller the number of subjects, the higher the risk of observing a larger number of adverse events in the vaccine arm. In other words, the smaller the number of subjects in the trial, the higher the likelihood of observing an anomalous result. Even one case could tilt the balance of the study. Every case of reported intussusception resulted in the entire team being extremely anxious, until the DSMB, after seeing the results (of whether the subject was in the placebo or vaccine group), cleared the study to continue recruiting.

The study design, the simulation of risk and the plan to monitor the safety of the subjects were presented to the VRBPAC of the FDA in May 2000. The committee unanimously approved the study design and provided guidance on a detailed monitoring plan for the parents/ legal guardians of the trial participants.

Finally, after all the planning and computer simulation to predict the potential risks, the study started. The first patient in the pivotal Phase III was dosed in January 2001. Extensive monitoring was required. Each subject was to be followed up with every six weeks by email, letters, telephone calls (this was the pre-mobile phone era), home visits and visits of the children to the clinics. Remember, the study covered 70,000 children in eleven countries. In addition, all the guardians of the children were trained on how to identify and report any stomach illness and signs and symptoms of intussusception. They were asked to report to the clinical study personnel within twenty-four hours of any incident. Diapers of the babies were regularly collected and shipped to the clinical sample management team in Wayne, Pennsylvania, where Joseph Kessler and Cheryl Moyer were coordinating entering the bar-coded diapers into the electronic system. Dan DiStefano, Fubao Wang, Laura Mallette and their teams at Merck had developed and validated a method to extract the DNA from the 'shit' (pardon the language) from the diapers, conduct a sophisticated polymerase chain reaction (PCR) test* and identify which strain of rotavirus was present. This method allowed the clinical data analytics team to determine whether vaccination was preventing rotavirus, the presence of which was detected by this method. Using this process, the success rate of follow-up (i.e. ability to find the patient again after the vaccine/placebo was administered) was 99.9 per cent, unprecedented for a study of this magnitude.

The DSMB plotted every case of intussusception on the continuous boundary of the monitoring graph and confirmed to the team that the vaccine was not causing an increased safety risk. It took four years to administer three doses of the vaccine or placebo to 60,000 subjects and collect all the clinical and laboratory data. But the process did not end after that. The DSMB required another 10,000 subjects to be enrolled because the study criteria had not

---

* Polymerase Chain Reaction (PCR) is a method to rapidly make millions to billions of copies of a specific DNA sample, allowing scientists to take a very small sample of DNA and amplify it. PCR was invented in 1983 by the American biochemist Kary Mullis at Cetus Corporation.

been met. Finally, in 2005, the study was unblinded, with 70,000 subjects. It was the largest clinical trial ever done. The goal of the trial was to ensure that the number of intussusception cases were equal in the vaccine and placebo groups, and not higher in the vaccinated group. With a huge sigh of relief, the statisticians reported that there were eleven cases of intussusception; five in the vaccine group and six in the placebo. The study passed its pre-defined criteria for a safe vaccine. It could not have been closer.

The REST trial was unique. The end point was a rare safety event. The innovative process of the continuous monitoring boundary graph, combined with a highly efficient clinical monitoring process, were the keys to success. A basic question when developing vaccines and drugs is how much safety data is enough? Generally, most vaccine trials have between 5000 and 10,000 subjects. The REST study compared 35,000 vaccine recipients to 35,000 placebo recipients. Is that enough? RotaShield® was given to nearly three million children in the first year. In order to ensure the safety of RotaTeq, post-approval safety studies were conducted. More than 1,69,000 children were monitored. There was no association of intussusception with the rotavirus vaccine.

Subsequently, GSK developed another vaccine to prevent rotavirus infections, called Rotarix®. The difference between the Merck and GSK vaccines is the backbone of the animal rotavirus strain that is used in the manufacture of the vaccines. Merck's vaccine is developed using the bovine rotavirus, and GSK uses a strain of rotavirus isolated from humans. Krishna Ella, who founded Bharat Biotech in India, developed another rotavirus vaccine, called Rotavac®, which is also made from a single isolate obtained from a human sample.

We started this chapter by asking why it costs so much to develop a vaccine. Vaccines are given predominantly to healthy individuals. Society does not accept any severe safety side effects in preventive vaccines. Hence even an extremely rare side effect of the rotavirus vaccine, despite its obvious large benefit of preventing deaths, is unacceptable. The rarer the side effect that needs to be studied, the larger the clinical trial and the higher the cost. Until there is an acceptance that all vaccines have some side effects, and their benefit outweighs the risks, society will struggle with the answer to these now often asked questions (during COVID-19 times): Which vaccine should I take? Is this vaccine safe? There are no perfect answers. The answer I generally give for the COVID-19 vaccines is, 'All the vaccines are equally unsafe'. The benefit of taking the vaccine far outweighs the risks of getting COVID-19-induced severe disease.

3

An Elusive Vaccine to Prevent AIDS

One of the biggest challenges of medicine.

The story of the discovery of the association of the human immunodeficiency virus (HIV) with the deadly disease AIDS (acquired immunodeficiency syndrome) is a fascinating and scandalous one for the field of science. American biomedical researcher Robert Gallo at the National Institutes of Health and French virologists Luc Montagnier and Françoise Barré-Sinoussi at the Pasteur Institute in Paris battled over the credit for making this seminal discovery. Both teams worked towards identifying the virus that causes this deadly disease. Discoveries in the fields of molecular biology, immunology and biochemistry were exploding thanks to the efforts to search for the mechanism by which the virus causes the disease. On 23 April 1984, when the world was listening to hits like *Hello* by Lionel Richie and watching movies like *Ghostbusters* and *Sharabi*, Gallo's team announced this monumental discovery through President Ronald Reagan's office. The then US Secretary of Health and Human Services announced that the vaccine against HIV would be available in two years. They could not have known how wrong they were. The French team was outraged, for they were the first to have discovered the virus. A public war over the right to the credit for the discovery ensued, with publications from both groups and investigative publications on the source of the discovery. Jon Cohen's book *Shots in the Dark*, and Randy Shilts's book *And the Band Played On: Politics, People and the AIDS Epidemic*, have the gory details. The discovery of the cause of AIDS and the subsequent war over the credit for this discovery involved hard work, deep science, deception, mystery, large egos and millions of dollars. Ultimately, the French scientists prevailed, and society recognized their accomplishment by awarding them the Nobel Prize in Physiology or Medicine in 2008. But this is just the tip of the iceberg of the fascinating story of one of the biggest challenges of mankind: to develop a vaccine against HIV.

The first decade (1980–90): Discovering the pathology of the disease and testing the envelope proteins of the virus as a vaccine

Back in the 1980s, HIV was causing widespread panic by killing people. In 1981, the *New York Times* reported forty-one cases of a rare type of cancer, called Kaposi sarcoma, in homosexual men.* It presents as huge purple patches on the skin. It is unmistakably visible. A mysterious illness causing bacterial infections in the lungs and fungal infections in the mouth was also reported in the *San Francisco Chronicle*. Patients were dying 'like flies'. This was a contemporary epidemic, not merely something one read about in history books (such as the Black Death, the bubonic plague in Europe that killed hundreds of millions of people between 1347 and 1351, or the 1918 influenza pandemic). Ironically, the world is now experiencing yet another pandemic, with the war on a microscopic virus equivalent to World War III.

The race to discover the source of the infection resulted in identifying the virus, HIV. It was killing the cells of the immune system, hence making patients susceptible to all possible infections and cancers. The US government poured resources into understanding the biology of this deadly virus. As a result, the 1980s saw an astoundingly large number of seminal discoveries in the field of immunology and virology. The receptor on immune cells that recognizes the virus, called the T cell receptor, was discovered by Canadian medical researcher Tak Wah Mak at the University of Toronto, Canada. Ellis Reinherz, working in Harvard, discovered specialized molecules in the immune cells, called CD4 (for cluster designation 4), which are expressed

---

* Altman, Lawrence K. 'Rare Cancer Seen in 41 Homosexuals', *New York Times*, 3 July 1981, Section A, p. 20.

on the major immune cells, aptly called CD4 T cells. In December 1984, Angus Dalgleish, a professor of oncology at St George's, University of London, and the team at the Chester Beatty Laboratories in London, made the pivotal discovery that the 120 kilodalton glycoprotein—gp120 protein*—of the virus binds specifically and precisely to the CD4 molecule on helper cells. They published the results of their work in the journal *Nature*. Voila! The scientists had defined the biology of the virus. The part of the virus that is responsible for entry into human cells was discovered (i.e., gp120); the cells it infects were identified (CD4 T cells); and the receptor through which HIV enters was defined (CD4 molecule).

I was then working at North Shore University Hospital–Cornell University Medical College, in the laboratory of Savita Pahwa. Originally from Delhi's Miranda House, she was an extremely kind and dedicated physician-scientist. The work I had done for my PhD (immunology of leprosy) and my meeting with Savita in the Taj Hotel in Mumbai were indeed my inflection points for my career. The following factors were important for that opportunity in my career progression: i) I had done my PhD on the development of a vaccine against leprosy under the guidance of Dr M.G. Deo and my mentor Rita Mulherkar,

---

* Gp120 is a specialized protein of the virus that makes up the envelope. 'Gp' stands for glycoprotein, where sugars (glycans) are attached to proteins, enabling them to have stable structures and bind efficiently to cells. 120 is the size of the glycoprotein (120 kilodalton).

and had thus learnt the basics of immunology; ii) Savita had been trained in clinical immunology on the art of bone marrow transplantation by Robert Good, the director of Memorial Sloan Kettering Institute in New York; iii) my good friend Naoki Oyaizu, a physician from Osaka, Japan, who had a deep understanding of the pathology of diseases who was my colleague; iv) handsome funding for doing the research on HIV pathogenesis from National Institutes of Health; v) an environment of creativity and exploration; vi) outstanding collaborators such as Carl Saxinger and V.S. Kalyanaraman; eminent scientists at the NIH in the field of HIV research at that time and vii) youth and energy.

It was not all smooth sailing. Competition, jealousy, favouritism, even the untimely death of colleagues, were all par for the course of a 'normal' new-job experience. The knowledge gained through our hard work prevailed, and we published extensively in peer-reviewed journals on various fundamental discoveries on the interaction of gp120 with the immune system that provided an understanding of pathogenesis of disease progression.

At that time, the vaccine developers hypothesized that an antibody to gp120 could block the binding of the virus to CD4 and prevent viral entry. That was how all the vaccines for various viruses had been successfully developed. The HIV gp120 envelope protein could be purified and injected into healthy volunteers. The immune response would develop antibodies to gp120, which would block the virus from binding to the CD4 receptor, block viral entry, and thus prevent AIDS. Simple! In 1984, US Secretary of Health and Human Services, Margaret Heckler, announced that a vaccine would be ready for testing in two years.[*]

Developing a vaccine was the obvious solution to preventing infection and containing the AIDS outbreak.[†] After all, the technology of developing successful vaccines was many decades old in the 1980s. Pharmaceutical companies had made vaccines against measles, mumps, rubella (MMR), diphtheria, pertussis, tetanus (DTP), polio and many other diseases. All these vaccines induced the immune system to generate antibodies, which in turn protected against infection by a particular bug. *How difficult could it be to develop a vaccine against HIV?* The process required involves developing a method to i) identify the major portion of the vaccine that induces protective immunity, which is the envelope glycoproteins; ii) removing all other components of the virus (such as the other proteins, the RNA); test it in monkeys to ensure its safety; and then test it in humans to confirm that it protects against infection. This process has been faithfully providing society with successful vaccines.

The purified gp120 protein was developed as a vaccine by Genentech. It was administered to subjects who were at high risk of getting infected. Hopes were extremely high

---

[*] Esparza, J. 'A Brief History of the Global Effort to Develop a Preventive HIV Vaccine'. *Vaccine*, 35 (2003): 3502–18.
[†] Cohen, J. *Shots in the Dark: The Wayward Search for an AIDS Vaccine*. WW Norton Publishers (2001).

in the AIDS community. The drama of these trials reached dizzying heights, with emerging biotechnology companies Genentech and Chiron spending millions to manufacture the product, and Daniel Zagury, a clinician-scientist from the Pierre and Marie Curie Institute in Paris, injecting himself with the vaccine. Everyone anxiously waited for the results. Finally, they were announced. The vaccine trials were dismal failures. The vaccine was unable to protect against the infection. Not only did it not prevent HIV infection, but the disease in the vaccinated individuals became more aggressive. It took a few years to discover the reason.

HIV is one of the most sophisticated products of the evolution of pathogens known to humans. The virus mutates extensively, thereby making millions of different strains. Each infected individual has many thousands of strains of the virus, each with a unique sequence of the gp120 protein, circulating in their body. A person is infected with the virus typically through sexual interactions or blood transfusions. The virus from the 'donor' enters the body of the 'recipient'. It infects CD4 positive cells by means of the gp120 portion of the virus binding specifically to CD4 molecules on T cells.[*] The virus replicates profusely. The immune system battles the virus-infected cells and

---

[*] Dalgleish, A.G., Beverley, P.C.L., Clapham, P.R., Crawford, D.H., Greaves, M.F. and Weiss, R.A. 'The CD4 (T4) Antigen is an Essential Component of the Receptor for the AIDS Retrovirus'. *Nature* 312, (1984): 763–67.

brings them under control by killing them. That is what the immune system has evolved to do. Following this attack by the immune system, the virus becomes dormant. It incorporates its genome into the chromosomes of the host. Here it remains silently, not expressing any protein or progeny virus. That is, the DNA of the virus is inserted into the host DNA (integrated), and the viral DNA is not making any protein of the virus. It is Silent. It is a reservoir for the future when the immune system becomes weak. Another strategy the virus uses is extensive mutations. The mutations are random. Those mutations that escape the attack of the immune system survive. These mutated HIV strains grow exponentially. The immune system is thus overwhelmed with mutated strains of the virus. The virus kills the CD4 T cells, which are central to the

PATHOGENESIS OF AIDS

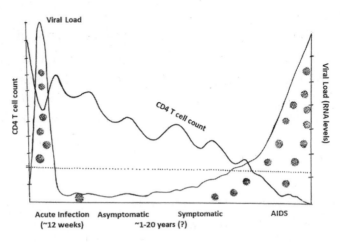

45

immune system. The patient now has no immune system and succumbs to various other bacterial infections.

So, how does one design a vaccine to block this complicated pathway of disease progression?

The gp120 vaccine, needed to induce the protective antibody response, would have to be made against each and every strain of HIV in an infected person. An impossible task. There are thousands of strains of the virus, each with a slightly different gp120 sequence. When the vaccine is given, the virus promptly mutates the gp120 sequence to a different sequence than that of the vaccine strain. The resulting strains, which escape the immune attack, are more virulent, making the disease worse. This 'standard' approach of developing a vaccine against an infectious pathogen was not going to work against HIV.

However, one of the most important attributes of scientists is mad persistence.

The second decade (1990–2000): Finding alternative ways to induce protective immunity against the virus; the radical discovery of chemical inhibitors of the virus

In 1998, at the University of Pennsylvania, Robert Doms made another remarkable discovery about the entry of HIV into CD4 T cells. It turns out that the CD4 molecule is only a decoy for the virus to enter the CD4 T cell. Gp120 on the virus binds to the CD4 molecule in step one of the entry process. In step two, gp120 detaches from the virus surface due to this interaction, thereby unveiling another protein under it, which is embedded in the membrane of the virus. This protein is called gp41. It interacts with another receptor on the CD4 T cells, called chemokine receptor type 5 (CCR5). Thus, the real culprit is gp41, the other envelope protein, which literally hides behind gp120 on the surface of the virus. Once gp120 is released (by binding to CD4), gp41 springs open with force and bores a hole in the T cell by interacting with CCR5.* This action of gp41 results in the fusion of the virus membrane with that of the T cell. The virus enters. This discovery changed the direction of vaccine development for HIV. Several scientists started studying the mechanism by which gp41 enters the cells and whether antibodies targeting this glycoprotein could block HIV infection. It was a sensational discovery. Many scientists started working on developing a vaccine using the virus protein that contains this gp41, called gp160. It was hypothesized that the gp160 protein vaccine should be able to induce antibodies that prevented entry of the virus.

Again, an army of scientists started developing these vaccines. Trials were initiated. Hopes were raised again. However, most of the trials, including large-scale Phase III trials by biopharmaceutical company VaxGen involving 5400 volunteers in the US and Netherlands, failed to meet their goal of inducing a protective immune response. It was

---

* Wilen, C.B., Tilton, J.C. and Doms, R.W. 'HIV: Cell Binding and Entry'. *Cold Spring Harbor Perspectives in Medicine* 2 (2011): a006866.

a dismal loss for the scientists. The reason was the same as that for gp120. The virus mutated away from the vaccine sequence.

Meanwhile, from 1990–2000, remarkable advances were being made in the area of small molecule chemical drugs that could kill the virus by binding to the most essential proteins that the virus requires for replication. The drugs targeted three classes of proteins of the virus. The first was the all-essential reverse transcriptase that converts the HIV viral genome (which is RNA) to DNA inside the cell. Azidothymine (AZT) was a very old drug that had been used to treat cancer. It specifically bound to the HIV reverse transcriptase. But giving the drug by itself was only a temporary cure. The virus's ability to mutate the genes responsible for AZT binding and retain the reverse transcriptase activity resulted in resistance to treatment. So, scientists discovered another molecule that blocked another important functional protein of the virus, the protease. The protease, as the name suggests, is an enzyme that digests certain proteins in the virus life cycle. During the process of protein production, a larger 'inactive' form is first made by cells. Subsequently, the large protein is 'cut' into smaller parts by protease enzymes. These multi-step processes are used by cells to be efficient and specific. This protease cleavage step is critical for HIV replication and development of the right active component made from larger proteins. A drug, such as Crixivan® made by Merck, that binds to the protease enzyme inhibits its enzymatic activity and cripples the virus. The next step was to target another enzyme of the virus, the integrase. This enzyme is required for the virus genome to integrate into that of the host. Without this step, it would not be possible for the virus to replicate since the virus is a parasite and uses the host support system to replicate. Killing these three critical steps blocks viral replication completely. The combination therapy has been instrumental in controlling disease progression in patients who are infected. The therapy is called highly active antiretroviral therapy: HAART.

I attended many international AIDS conferences in the 1990s in Durban, Barcelona, Montreal, San Francisco and Washington DC. The conferences were focused on sharing knowledge of the science of the disease. Over the years, they became unique forums where science, public policy and human rights intersected. These interactions helped in the process of finding better treatment options for patients, increasing awareness of the disease, and putting a human face to the science of the disease.

At that time, the AIDS epidemic in India was just beginning. The epidemic's epicentre was in the northeast, where there was widespread intravenous drug use with shared needles. It soon spread throughout the country. The drugs used in the combination therapy were hard to come by since they were not available in India. Cipla, the pharmaceutical company headed by Yusuf Hamied, made significant advances in manufacturing the drugs used in the treatment of HIV at a fraction of the cost—at $1 a day, rather than $400. But fierce battles on intellectual property rights by pharmaceutical companies ensued. WHO and the Bill and Melinda Gates Foundation, supported the cause of making affordable drugs for the world. Cipla prevailed.*

Drugs for the treatment of HIV are now approved and their availability has made it possible for AIDS patients in India to live longer lives. These drugs have to be taken every day. Stopping treatment results in reactivation of the virus, progression to AIDS and death. The drugs have a lot of toxic side effects. They are not able to eliminate the reservoir of cells that harbour the HIV genome; the cells that are dormant, quietly waiting for an opportunity to replicate when the drugs are not in circulation. The drugs are not a cure. They do not prevent infection. Prevention requires a vaccine.

The third decade (2000–10): It's the T cell, stupid

The scientific community developing a vaccine against HIV was at their wits' end. They needed a miracle. Bruce Walker, a physician-scientist at Harvard Medical School, found one.

Before we dive into this fascinating story of the HIV vaccine, we need to understand the complexities of the

---

* McNeil, D.G. Jr. 'Selling Cheap "Generic" Drugs, India's Copycats Irk Industry'. *New York Times*, (2000).

immune system. The immune system is the body's armed forces. It is educated (trained) by the 'universities' (the bone marrow and thymus) of the body. After this training, the cells of the immune system patrol the body through its circulatory system and look for foreign agents. When they identify the agent (for example, a virus or bacteria), they attack the bug and kill it. The army of the immune system is made up of two major brigades: the cell-mediated immune system and the humoral immune system. The former is the infantry and the latter the air force.

The cell-mediated immune system comprises CD8 T cells, which can kill infected cells (such as the HIV-infected cells) in hand-to-hand combat by puncturing holes in them and injecting lethal proteins (missiles) into them. The CD8 T cells recognize the infected cells with very specialized equipment (receptors), which sends signals to activate the missile system (perforins and granzymes), which make pores in the target cells and kill them. The molecules (receptors) on the CD8 killer cells bind to the virus on infected cells, and this recognition interaction is important for the specificity, so that they do not kill non-infected cells indiscriminately.

On the other hand, the B cells of the humoral system, when activated by receptors that recognize a foreign agent, can secrete antibodies directed against viruses and bacteria. These antibodies travel long distances through the circulatory system and hunt down foreign agents with precision and accuracy.

There is one other very important component of the immune system, the CD4 T cells. These cells are the all-important controllers of both the cell-mediated and humoral immune systems. Just like a nuclear reactor requires at least two keys to be activated, both CD8 T cells and B cells require help from the CD4 T cells. These helper CD4 T cells secrete growth factors that provide signals to the CD8 T and B cells to kill and secrete antibodies, respectively, against the invading virus or bacteria. HIV kills the CD4 T cells, thus paralysing the immune system at the core.

Most vaccines developed today activate the humoral immune system, which results in the development of antibodies, which in turn prevent the virus from entering cells.

Now back to our story of combating HIV.

The pathogenesis of the disease with respect to viral replication was being unveiled through the vaccine studies. Everyone who was infected with HIV had one strain of the virus in the early phase of the disease. The immune system was extremely efficient in eliminating the majority (most importantly, not all) of the virus from circulation. The remaining virus then went dormant for many years. Today, patients are treated with a cocktail of drugs, which control the virus's growth and thereby control progression to the symptoms of AIDS. However, the virus is mutating constantly, slowly replicating into various versions of itself. This is the mechanism by which it escapes the attack by the immune system. Ultimately, there is sufficient mass

**THE PLAYERS
OF SOCIETY**

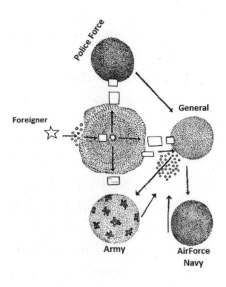

**THE PLAYERS
OF THE IMMUNE SYSTEM**

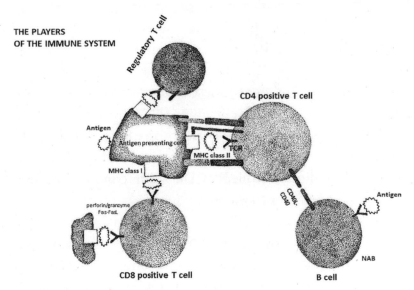

Antigen presenting cells (such as dendritic cells), CD4+ T helper cells, CD8+ cytotoxic T cells, antibody secreting B cells and regulatory T cells are shown above.

of the mutated viruses, which attack the immune system viciously, and the person succumbs to the disease.

As the results of the dismal failures of the clinical trials using the envelope proteins as vaccines were being reported, a very interesting new story involving unexplained protection against the virus in humans was emerging from an unlikely source. There were some sex workers in West Africa who, despite having had sex with several partners infected with HIV, did not develop the symptoms of AIDS. They were infected with the virus, but there was something about their immune system that prevented the virus from reproducing and replicating. Bruce Walker of the Harvard Medical School was systematically studying the immune systems of these sex workers. He discovered that these women, after sexual encounters, had very high levels of CD8 T cells. The killer cells. He hypothesized that the higher number of these killer cells were killing the HIV-infected cells and curtailing HIV from replicating. There was a strong inverse correlation of high CD8 T cells that recognized the virus, with viral load. He called these individuals 'elite controllers'. CD8 T cells comprise another 'wing' of the immune system.

Many more reports from various parts of the world started flooding the literature with this characteristic of the disease. Those who got infected with HIV but did not have clinical disease symptoms of multiple infections and cancers were aptly called long-term non-progressors (LTNP). Their immune systems could control

HIV without affecting CD4 T cell loss, without the need for any anti-HIV medicines. More studies done by Dan Barouch and Norman Letvin, professors of medicine at Harvard Medical School, in rhesus monkeys showed that CD8 T cells were critical in controlling HIV replication. They depleted the CD8 T cells in monkeys by treating them with a CD8 T antibody, which resulted in a very aggressive form of HIV. Several other researchers were making the same observations, that activation of the CD8 T cell was crucial in the protective immune response against HIV. The wave of the field drifted from humoral immune responses to cell-mediated immune responses.

However, it is not easy to activate the CD8 T cell-mediated immune system.

To understand why, let's go back to some more basics of the immune system and something called antigen presentation. Bacteria and viruses evolved several millions of years ago and have been co-evolving with humans ever since the first Homo sapiens arrived. The major difference between a bacterium and a virus is that the former can replicate by itself, i.e., it has all the components of reproduction—from DNA to the enzymes—to duplicate itself. A virus, on the other hand, has its own DNA or RNA, but utilizes the machinery of the host cell, the enzymes and organelles, to divide. It is thus a parasite. The cells of the immune system have also evolved along with these single-cell organisms. Bacteria are 'eaten' by macrophages, specialized cells that engulf foreign agents.

They chop up the bacteria into smaller parts (peptides) in the lysosome, an organelle filled with digestive enzymes. A flagging protein, called the human leukocyte antigen type 2 (HLA2), binds to this bacterial peptide and 'presents it' on the surface of the macrophage. Now, this macrophage is 'displaying' to the immune system that it has been infected with the bacteria. CD4 T cells, which have a receptor that recognizes the bacterial peptide presented by HLA2, are activated and in turn start to secrete activating proteins (cytokines). These cytokines then activate B cells, which make antibodies to the bacteria. The antibodies hunt down the free flying bacteria in the body and kill them. This is the mechanism by which the humoral immune response is triggered. It is the process that all vaccines use to activate the immune system. In the case of vaccines, instead of the bacterium itself, a small portion of the bacterium is utilized.

Viruses, however, are a different beast. When a virus enters a cell, it uses a clever way to transport its DNA or RNA to the nucleus of the cell. For it is here that all the necessary machinery for replication is present—the enzymes for dividing the DNA (nucleotides) and rich nutrients. The virus divides. But wait. The immune system has also intelligently countered the virus's sneaky entry. When the viral protein is produced inside the cellular machinery, like all other proteins, the cell transports the viral protein to the endoplasmic reticulum, a long tube-like structure inside the cell where proteins get 'dressed' before they exit the cell. Here another flag protein, called HLA1, binds to the new virus peptides that are present in the endoplasmic reticulum. These HLA1-bound virus peptides are 'presented' on the surface of the cell and are recognized by CD8 'killer' T cells. CD8 T cells are thus activated, which triggers them to release proteins (perforins) and enzymes (granzymes) that make pores in virus-infected cells and kill them. This process of activating the CD8 T cells is known as cell-mediated immunity.

So, if the immune system is so good at killing virus-infected cells with CD8 T cells, why does one get AIDS? An additional nuance of the activation of B cells (humoral immunity) and CD8 T cells (cell-mediated immunity) is that both require help from CD4 T cells. Without this help, neither can be activated. Since HIV kills CD4 T cells, it cripples the immune system. This process is the essence of the mechanism of the path from HIV infection to the development of AIDS.

A vaccine should be able to kill virus-infected cells. In 2000, scientists at Merck, led by Emilio Emini and John Shiver, hypothesized that if a CD8 T cell specific to the HIV protein can be activated prior to the first infection by HIV, the immune system should be able to kill virus-infected cells before large amounts of the virus can grow. The goal of the vaccine then was to activate HIV-specific CD8 T cells through vaccination and induce immunological memory to HIV.

In order to understand the design of this innovative vaccine, we need to discuss the adenovirus, a virus that causes the common cold. This virus has a DNA material that enables the virus to replicate inside the cells of our bodies. The DNA of this virus was genetically engineered (i.e., DNA is cut using enzymes and molecular engineering techniques) and replaced with the DNA of a small portion of HIV proteins (called gag, pol and nef, or GPN). These GPN HIV proteins by themselves cannot make a full virus since thirteen different proteins are required to make an infectious virus. The adenovirus-virus expressing the HIV GPN proteins (this virus is now called a 'vector' since it is transporting the HIV GPN proteins to the cells) is injected as a vaccine. It inserts its DNA into the nucleus of the cell, like all viruses do. Since it is HIV protein DNA, the cell makes these HIV proteins, which bind to HLA1 in the endoplasmic reticulum and present as a flag on the surface of these cells. CD8 T cells, which specifically recognize foreign agents when presented by HLA1, get activated. Since there is no HIV circulating, the CD8 T cells just multiply and get ready. These are memory CD8 T cells. When a person is infected with HIV, the HIV proteins are also presented on the surface by HLA1, flagging these cells as HIV-infected cells. The activated memory cells hunt down these HIV-infected cells and kill them. The hypothesis that inducing activation of CD8 T cells to protect from HIV-infected cells was supported by the observations from the study of the immune systems of the West African sex workers and the studies conducted using monkeys. That CD8 T cells were required and sufficient for protection against HIV infection and AIDS was the 'KoolAid' that everyone was drinking.

It was time to test this hypothesis. The planning of the clinical trial started at Merck in West Point, Pennsylvania. Several scientists at Merck, advisers from the National Institutes of Health and many clinicians from across the world (Thailand, Malawi, Boston, Seattle and twenty different institutions) came together and designed one of the more interesting clinical trials in infectious disease vaccines. It was christened the STEP trial.* † It was not an acronym. It was also called Merck V520 Protocol 023, Phambili in Africa and HVTN 503 at the National Institutes of Health. The study design involved giving healthy volunteers either the adenovirus-GPN vaccine or the placebo. The study was blind, such that neither the person who administered the vaccine not the recipient of the vaccine knew whether that individual had received the vaccine or a placebo. Since the subjects chosen for the study were at high risk of getting infected with HIV due to their promiscuous behaviour, there were many folks who were infected during the course

* Sekaly, R.P. 'The Failed HIV Merck Vaccine Trial: a Step Back or Future Launching Point for Future Vaccine Development?'. *Journal of Experimental Medicine*, 205 (2008): 7–12.

† Gray, G., Buchbinder, S. and Duerr, A. 'Overview of STEP and Phambili Trial Results: Two Phase IIb Test-of-Concept Studies Investigating the Efficacy of MRK Adenovirus Type 5 gag/pol/nef subtype B HIV Vaccine'. *Curr. Opin HIV AIDS* 5 (2010): 357–61.

of the trial. The hypothesis was that the same number of people got infected, in both vaccinated, and placebo groups, and the vaccinated individuals would clear the virus since they would have activated CD8 killer T cells. The result was the most dramatic in the history of vaccines. More people got infected with HIV if they were vaccinated, compared to the placebo-treated individuals. Forty-nine of the 914 men in the vaccine group, and thirty-three of the 922 men in the placebo group tested positive for HIV. The trial was stopped. In May 2012, the *New York Times* reported that the vaccine given to volunteers made them more and not less likely to be infected with HIV.*

How was it that such a disaster had not been anticipated? Basic immunology teaches us that in order to activate the CD8 T killer cells, help from CD4 T cells is required. *Which cells did the vaccine activate?* The HIV-specific, activated CD4 T cells. *Which cells does HIV like to infect?* The HIV-specific, activated CD4 T cells. The adenovirus-GPN vaccine induced an increase in the number of these cells and created an infectable reservoir for HIV. This may be the most plausible explanation for the results of the STEP trial. Many scientists involved with the study have given many different hypotheses for the anomalous result, but the stark reality was staring the HIV vaccine developers in the face.

---

* Altman, L. 'Trial for Vaccine against H.I.V. is Canceled'. *New York Times* (2008).

It was another calamity in the field. The scientists were looking for another miracle. And it came.

The fourth decade (2010–20): Developing broadly neutralizing antibodies

An interesting result was observed in a vaccine trial, called RV144, being conducted by the National Institutes of Health in Thailand.* The vaccine being tested with a combination of another vector AL-VAC, made from a virus that infects canarypox birds (but not humans), along with a second different vaccine which comprised injections of the envelope glycoprotein gp120. In this trial, where volunteers were either vaccinated or given a placebo, the vaccinated group showed a 31 per cent protection rate, which was a modest rate. The findings discovered while understanding the mechanism of protection pointed to the importance of antibody responses. More importantly, antibodies that have a specific function, called antibody-dependent cellular cytotoxicity. It is a process by which certain cells of the immune system (not the professional CD8 killer T cells), such as neutrophils, can become killers when an antibody to the virus attaches to them through a receptor called the Fc receptor. Furthermore, the vaccine

---

* Karasavvas, N. et al. 'The Thai Phase III HIV Type 1 Vaccine Trial (RV144) Regimen Induces Antibodies that Target Conserved Regions within the V2 Loop of gp120'. *AIDS Research and Human Retroviruses*, 28 (2012): 1444–57.

also elicited a much weaker CD4 T helper cell response, which was necessary for the B cells to secrete HIV envelope-specific antibodies. The results of this trial revolutionized the thinking in the industry.

With the availability of sophisticated technologies for identifying the structures of proteins, American scientist Peter Kim at the Massachusetts Institute of Technology (MIT) was studying how HIV enters the cell through its interactions with CD4 and CCR5 proteins on CD4 T cells. A structural biologist, he developed methods to reveal the structure of the portion of the virus envelope where gp120 interacts with gp41 (which is tethered to the virus membrane). As we have seen, gp120 binds to CD4 molecules on CD4 T cells and is removed, exposing the gp41 region. The gp41 protein is like a tightly coiled spring when gp120 'sits' on its head. Once the gp120 separates, 'twang' like a spring, it forces open, boring through the membrane of the CD4 T cells. This process allows the membrane of the virus to fuse with the membrane of the CD4 T cells. The virus then unloads its cargo—the viral RNA—into the cell. The RNA enters the nucleus and through a process of reverse transcription, followed by integration, infects the host. When the host cell divides, millions of virus particles are made. This is the process of virus entry and replication. The fusion of the gp41 region with the membrane of the cell is a universal process, in that every strain of HIV utilizes the same mechanism. If the virus tries to mutate this sequence, that strain of the virus loses its infectability and it dies. Thus, this is the hot spot on the envelope protein against which the vaccine should be developed.

How was it that extensive research by thousands of scientists working for more than three decades was not able to define this hot spot as the weak link of the virus and develop a vaccine? It was not easy.

The envelope glycoprotein is expressed as a trimeric form (i.e., three molecules of the envelope are associated with each other), which shields the region that is broadly neutralizing and prevents antibodies from binding to that site. Broadly neutralizing antibodies are defined by their ability to block entry of all the strains of HIV.[*] The neutralizing site on the envelope is the most critical domain for the virus to enter CD4+ cells.

Interestingly, many studies have isolated such antibodies that bind to the protected site. However, these antibodies form much later in the disease progression, at which point it is too late to protect the immune cells from being destroyed. The positive factors are that since such broadly neutralizing antibodies arise during natural infections, and these antibodies have been demonstrated to block the infection by multiple strains of HIV in animal experimental studies, it should be possible to develop a vaccine targeting this domain of the envelope.

---

[*] Sok, D. and Haynes, B.R. 'Recent Progress in Broadly Neutralizing Antibodies to HIV'. *Nature Immunology* 19 (2018): 1179–88.

So, what is this domain that is protected so arduously by the virus? How does it prevent the immune system from developing effective antibodies? Let us try and understand how this domain of the envelope works.

The infection of the cell by HIV starts by entry of the virus through binding of the envelope glycoprotein gp120 (explained earlier) to CD4 molecules on T cells. These cells also express the co-receptor CCR5, which is required for the virus to enter the cells. The gp120 protein acts in threes (trimers) (see figure on the next page). The first interaction of gp120 with CD4 results in separation of the gp120 from the surface of the virus envelope, revealing the gp41 portion. The other portion of gp120 (called variable loop [V3]) (see figure on the next page) binds to the co-receptor CCR5, and brings the two membranes together. The domain in gp41 is like a compressed spring. When gp120 is removed, the gp41 'spring' opens out like a jack-in-the-box and creates a pore in the T cell. The process results in the fusion of the two membranes, which then enables the virus to release its payload, the viral RNA, into the cell, infecting it.

Thus, to block the virus from entry, the immune system needs to develop an antibody that binds to the gp41 domain of the virus *after* the spring has opened. A very difficult and formidable task. That portion of the gp41 is opened only for a few milliseconds. The antibody should be present in high enough concentrations to block this interaction. There is also the physical constraint that the antibody molecule is

HIV ENTRY

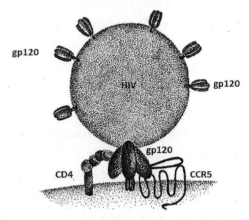

Schematic diagram of viral entry: The virus attaches to the host cells via the viral envelope protein gp120 that binds to the surface of the CD4 molecules (1). This interaction causes a conformational change in the envelope, which enables the V3 loop to bind to CCR5 (2). The actions stabilize the interaction bringing the two membranes towards each other. This binding exposes the gp41 domain and initiates the membrane fusion process through the trimer peptides of gp41 inducing a pore and resulting in membrane fusion.

very large (150 kilodaltons) and does not fit easily into the space between the membrane of the virus and CD4+ T cell when the fusion is occurring. Making an antibody to the non-sprung gp41 is not effective since this is not the portion of the virus that is required for viral entry.

The year was 2012. I was invited to be a member of the NIH's advisory committee to review proposals for funding thanks to a recommendation by my good friend Annie DeGroot. Annie is the CEO of EpiVax, a company dedicated to using data analytics to identify the active components of vaccines and biologics through an innovative computer algorithm. She and I share a common interest in understanding the pathogenesis of HIV. I was selected based on my credentials of almost two decades of experience in studying the pathogenesis of HIV, and probably more importantly, being part of the team that experienced the failed HIV vaccine STEP trial.

The selection of members of such advisory committees is a very detailed process. It is an honour to be selected, and a consequence of a lifetime of experience on a specific subject. The committee comprises about ten experts hailing from different disciplines. The grant applications are sent to the review committee several months in advance. Each grant application has a specific aim, background, preliminary results that support the aims, experimental design, anticipated results, and a concept note on impact to the field. NIH funding has helped enable extremely innovative and high-risk-of-failure hypotheses. It is very likely that almost every major innovation in the field of biological science has benefitted from NIH funding. It is a mechanism of funding with a very low return on investment and net present value, which industry will rarely venture.

The committee sent out a request for proposals for extending the results from the RV144 study for NIH funding. Seven major scientific teams' proposals were funded. All of them focused on the development of vaccines to induce broadly reactive neutralizing antibodies directed at the gp120-gp41 hinge region of the virus, the hot spot that was critical for the entry of the virus into the cell. If a vaccine could elicit an immune response that made antibodies to this region of the envelope, viral entry should be prevented. A vaccine was in sight.

The seven proposals were all top secret. These are ideas that are proposed to revolutionize the field and cannot be shared. They lead to Nobel Prizes. Confidentiality is sworn and legally enforced by signatures. However, once the work funded by an NIH grant is published, it is in the public domain. I am now able to list some of the fantastic ideas that the grants proposed.

So, how does one develop broadly neutralizing antibodies for a portion of the virus that is hidden by a trimer of the envelope, expressed for only milliseconds, and that need to be present in high enough concentrations in a physically very tight space between the membranes of the virus and cell? The various grant proposals defined the portions of the envelope that, if attacked by an antibody, render the virus vulnerable. These areas fall in seven categories: i) the CD4 binding site (i.e. the portion of the CD4 molecule on the T cells that the viral envelope, gp120 binds to); ii) the virus membrane proximal external region (the external facing portion of the viral envelope, gp120); iii) the glycan patch (i.e. the sugar molecules that are associated with the viral envelope, gp120); iv) the tip of the V3 loop (a portion of the viral envelope gp120, that is named as the third variable loop to which antibodies can bind); v) the trimer dependent epitope at the apex of the envelope spike (the viral envelope protein always interacts with the CD4 molecules in multiples of threes (trimer), which allows the conformational folding of the two proteins to interact); vi) the interface between gp120 and gp41 (the portion between the gp120 [external facing part of the viral envelope] and gp41 [the internal portion of the viral envelope, that is bound to the viral membrane]); and vii) specific glycan and fusion peptide at the N terminal of gp41 (the protein and sugar molecules of gp41, that get exposed after gp120 is removed, by binding to the CD4 molecule). To completely block the ability of the envelope to mediate entry of the virus into the cell, all seven components of the envelope need to be neutralized. This is the huge challenge for vaccinologists to solve.

To elicit broadly neutralizing antibodies, the immune system needs to be challenged with a sequential immunization protocol of all the seven components listed above in a precisely orchestrated process. This schedule of vaccination would require a large study to account for the mutations that occur during the evolution of the virus, using the assumption that antibodies directed against the portions of the viral envelope protein, gp120, make the virus vulnerable. Each vaccinated person would respond to the vaccine differently, and therefore developing a generalized process of the vaccination schedule requires a study to monitor the progress of the antibody responses generated until such time that a broadly neutralizing antibody repertoire is achieved. This protocol will require a large clinical trial and a systematic study of the evolution of antibodies over time, followed by a clinical assessment to determine whether the antibodies indeed protect against HIV infection. A study of this nature will take another decade. But this is the pace of discovering the elusive vaccine against HIV.

Thus, to summarize the overall strategy, the challenge in developing a neutralizing antibody to the gp41 is to develop the well-ordered soluble trimer that faithfully represents the envelope on the surface of the virus. Just making the soluble protein has not been sufficient to develop the broadly neutralizing antibodies in animal models. The RV144 trial, which used a two dose regimen, consisting of an initial dose (called prime) followed by a second dose (called booster)—prime boost—regimen of canarypox virus expressing env, gag and protease genes, followed by a boost with soluble gp120, provided modest protection against preventing HIV infection. The vaccine also induced a mild cytotoxic killer T cell response in the vaccinated individuals. It is this combination of broadly neutralizing antibodies and a cytolytic T cell response that will be required to develop a vaccine that will prevent HIV infection. Time will tell whether this hypothesis is proven.

4

The Story of Immunotherapy

A possibility of a cure for some cancers.

The concept that the immune system can control cancers was proposed at the turn of the twentieth century by German scientists Wilhelm Busch and Friedrich Fehleisen, who were working at the University of Würzburg. In the 1860s, they intentionally injected Streptococcus bacteria (which causes a skin rash) into several patients' tumours, which induced the tumours to shrink and led to complete remission for several types of cancers. American bone surgeon and cancer researcher William B. Coley in 1891 systematically studied this process and injected cancer tissues with Staphylococcus bacterial cultures. The patients survived for more than eight years.[*]

---

[*] Dobosz, P. and Dzieciatkowski, T.J. 'The Intriguing History of Cancer Immunotherapy'. *Frontiers in Immunology* 10 (2019): 2965, 1–10.

The next major milestone in immunotherapy came in the mid-1980s. Cancer researcher and surgeon Steven Rosenberg at the National Cancer Institute at NIH treated patients with cell therapy by removing immune cells from the tumour infiltrating lymphocyte cells (Tumour infiltrating lymphonyces [TILs]), culturing them in the laboratory and reinjecting them into the patient. This treatment showed some efficacy.

The beginning of the 1980s was a revolutionary time in the field of immunology. I was studying for my PhD at the Cancer Research Institute, in Parel in 1982. We often held journal club meetings where we discussed the findings by Steven Rosenberg with great interest. Extensive discussions over cutting chai with my dear friends Robin Mukhopadhyay, Shyam Somasundaram, Satyamoorthy and many others allowed us to learn the importance of conducting detailed research to understand the complex science of the immunology of cancer. Shyam, who worked on basic aspects of cancer immunotherapy at the Wistar Institute in Philadelphia for more than thirty years, passed away in February 2021. We are still reconciling ourselves to this loss.

With the advent of the 'new disease' AIDS in the 1980s, there was a dire need to understand the components and workings of the immune system. Seminal discoveries about the immune system were made by studying HIV pathogenesis. Interleukin-2 (IL-2) was discovered at NIH by Doris Morgan, Francis Ruscetti and Robert Gallo.

IL-2 is a protein made by a specialized group of white blood cells, called helper T cells (also called CD4 positive T cells), which are responsible for expanding the immune army of the body. Some T cells differentiate into killer cells, called CD8 positive cytotoxic T cells, which can kill tumour cells and virus-infected cells of our body. Both CD4 and CD8 T cells require IL-2 to be activated to do their jobs. Rosenberg conducted several trials using IL-2 therapy with Cetus Corporation in California (in later years, Chiron purchased Cetus and Novartis bought Chiron). IL-2 was not consistently successful in treating patients with cancer. Some patients benefited, others displayed no effect, and a few also experienced a worsening of the disease. Clearly, the complex process of the regulation of the immune system was far from understood in the 1980s.

The basic concepts of the immune system that are taught in biology class in undergraduate courses these days show how much progress has been made in this field in a short span of thirty years. Antigens (which are parts of organisms that can activate the immune system) are processed by antigen presenting cells (APCs) as small bits of proteins (called peptides) to T cells. T cells recognize these peptides that are 'presented' to the immune system by molecules on APCs called major histocompatibility complex (MHC). The T cell receptors (TCR) on T cells recognize the MHC–peptide antigen complex and deliver 'signal one' for activation. The signal comprises the activation of a series of enzymes in the cell, called kinases. These kinases convert the energy molecule adenosine triphosphate (ATP) to adenosine diphosphate (ADP), release a phosphorus molecule, which in turn activates other enzymes. This cascade is termed as a 'signal'. Edmond Fischer and Edwin Krebs were awarded the Nobel Prize in Physiology or Medicine in 1992 for their pioneering work in describing the molecular basis of signal transduction.

The year was 1980. The Cold War was on. The US navy had placed battleships near the Soviet coasts and the Sea of Japan, anticipating nuclear threats. Carl June and Craig Thompson, physicians at the US Naval Medical School in Washington, D.C., were sent to Fred Hutchinson Cancer Research Center in Seattle to learn the process of bone marrow transplantation (BMT) since it was the one therapy that would be able to treat soldiers who may be exposed to nuclear radiation. BMT was being developed to treat patients with leukaemia. The experiments that Carl and Craig performed at Fred Hutch revolutionized the field. While BMT had some successes (pioneered by the work of Edward Donnall Thomas in Seattle and Robert Good at the Sloan Kettering Institute in New York), it was observed that some patients developed graft-versus-host disease (a violent immune rejection of the bone marrow by the host's immune system), which resulted in a horrific death. In fact, the BMT-induced graft-versus-host disease death was worse than the cancer itself. Patients were being treated with very harsh chemical drugs, which could suppress the graft-versus-host disease, but which had terrible side effects such as nausea, vomiting, lung and liver problems and weakness due to muscle wasting. It was then that cyclosporine A, a drug that was isolated in 1971 from a fungus called *Tolypocladium inflatum* by scientists from Sandoz (now Novartis) was discovered. Cyclosporine A was an immunosuppressant—it was able to suppress the immune system without major side effects in animal studies. Thomas Starzl at the University of Pittsburgh and Roy Yorke Calne at the University of Cambridge were doing work to understand the clinical use of the drug to suppress the immune system for kidney and liver transplantation.

That immune suppression was required for a successful transplant was established with the experiments done with cyclosporine A. Many other immunosuppressive drugs began to be developed, and the molecular and cellular mechanisms by which they inhibited the immune system began to be understood. One such mechanism involved a molecule on T cells called CD28. It is a molecule that is critical for T cell activation. The precise mechanism by which it induces T cell activation is where the story of our protagonist Dr Carl June's work on cell therapy for cancer begins.

Carl June and his colleagues also tested cyclosporine A for preventing graft-versus-host disease in BMT patients. It was extremely efficient in suppressing T cell responses. The scientists at Fred Hutch had made a new antibody called 9.3.* This antibody had an unusual function.

---

* June, C.H., Ledbetter, J., Linsley, P. and Thompson, C. 'Role of the CD28 Receptor in T-cell Activation'. *Immunology Today* 11 (1990): 211–6.

While cyclosporine A could suppress T cell functions extremely efficiently, the addition of the 9.3 antibody into the T cell culture overcame the suppression of cyclosporine. Yes, this is a confusing result. Hence there needed to be a systematic (forensic) approach to decipher the function of this protein. It turned out that the 9.3 antibody recognized that molecule on T cells, CD28. It had an unusual function. Stimulating T cells through the CD28 molecule by itself did not activate them, but sequential stimulation, first through the T cell receptor, and then CD28, was crucial for optimal stimulation of these cells. While a few other folks had been searching for such a molecule, it took a team of scientists with diverse experiences to find it. Indeed, ingenious minds that can think of remarkable experiments, when unexpected observations are observed. Carl June and his colleagues had inadvertently found a super-activator of T cells. They hypothesized that activation of T cells with anti-CD28 antibodies could activate the immune system in cancer patients, who generally had very suppressed immune responses. After completing their training, Carl June and Craig Thompson went back to the Naval Medical School in Washington, D.C. The Cold War had ended and defence funding was diverted to more important issues such as combating HIV and malaria. Carl June's research would now focus on these diseases, and it would take another decade before his ground-breaking research on Chimeric Antigen Receptor-T cells (CAR-T cells) would be used to treat cancer. We shall see how the CD28 story relates to these cells a bit later.

These complex concepts may well be confusing to the reader. T cell receptor, CD3, cyclosporine A, 9.3, CD28. Immunology jargon. To explain this biology, let us revisit some of the basic principles of immunology.

Let us use the analogy of a terrorist attacking a city to understand how a killer T cell kills its target. The two processes are quite similar. A terrorist enters the municipal headquarters of the city with the intention to hold the mayor and staff hostage and lay siege to the city. The smart receptionist asks for and distributes the business card of the terrorist to various departments of the mayor's office. Among those who get the business card are the police and the mayor. When the mayor sees the business card, it is immediately obvious that the terrorist has a history of crimes and has evil intent. However, due to the rules of civilized society, the mayor cannot act to eliminate the terrorist based on just one piece of information. Subsequently, the police do a background check and inform the mayor that the terrorist has weapons and has a gang working with him, and that they intend to cause harm. This second piece of information confirms that the terrorist is bad and needs to be eliminated. But by this time, it's too late. The terrorist and his gang have invaded the city. The mayor summons the armed forces. The general of the armed forces takes charge and gives orders to attack the invaders. The various groups of the armed forces act as they have been trained.

Ultimately, the bombs and missiles of the air force and navy as well as hand-to-hand combat by the army destroy and obliterate the terrorists. Peace is restored.

The terrorist is the tumour cell. The receptionist is a specialized white blood cell, called antigen presenting cell (APC), such as a dendritic cell. The police are regulatory T cells, and the CD4 helper is the mayor and then the general of the armed forces. B cells, which secrete antibodies, are the army and navy, the killer T cells are the army, which kill their targets in hand-to-hand combat (refer to figure on page 78). The technical description of the process is described below for the advanced reader.

The interface between the APC and T cell is called an 'immunological synapse' (much like that of a neuron in the brain). Several molecules are involved in this interaction including the T cell receptor molecule, which recognizes the antigen, the CD3 molecule (which has a long tail through the cell membrane and transduces the biochemical phosphorylation signal), the CD4 molecule, which binds to the MHC molecule on APC, adhesion molecules LFA-1 and ICAM-1 and many others. The interactions of these molecules on T cells with their specific partners on the APC are like a zip on a dress. One mismatch and the entire zip falls apart.

Specific binding of the processed antigen (the business card of the terrorist) delivers a signal to the CD4 T helper cell. This first signal, signal one, activates these cells by upregulating other molecules, mainly CD40 ligand.

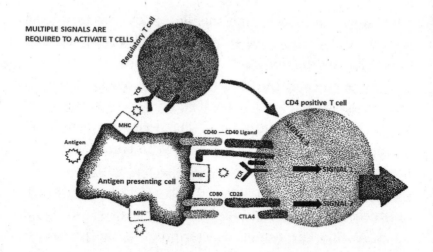

CD40 ligand bind to CD40 on APC, which in turn upregulate another set of molecules, CD80 and CD86 molecules. This cascading activation of cells and upregulation of molecules is the mechanism by which the immune system regulates the activation of T cells, ensures specific activation (non-specific activation can lead to T cells killing the body's own cells, i.e. autoimmunity), and enables an exponential expansion of the immune cells. The CD80 and CD86 molecules on antigen presenting cells, are the molecules that bind to CD28 on T cells and delivers signal two. This signal two combined with signal one, are the two switches for activating a T cell to respond to the foreign antigen. Much like the activation of a nuclear reactor requires at least two independent keys, so does the activation of the immune system. Once activated, it unleashes its immense power to eliminate the invader.

The activation of T cells results in the secretion of several growth factors such as IL-2, interferon gamma (IFNγ) and interleukin 4 (IL-4). This two-signal model of T cell activation was studied and defined by Ronald Schwartz at the NIH. Blocking the signal cascade by using an anti-CD4 antibody, an anti-CD40L antibody, or an anti-CD28 antibody results in blocking T cell activation. This concept was very important for blocking overly active T cells that cause autoimmune diseases, where activated T cells attack cells in the organs of the body, such as pancreas (autoimmune diabetes), brain (multiple sclerosis), muscle (myasthenia gravis) and others. Blocking T cell activation could ameliorate autoimmunity. On the other hand, using an anti-CD28 antibody to activate the T cell without the need for signal one through the T cell receptor-CD3 receptors could be very useful for the treatment of cancer patients. The antibody was the drug that was tested.

The drug, which was manufactured by TeGenero Pharmaceutical, was known as theralizumab or TGN14134. It was developed by Professor Thomas Hünig at the University of Würzburg. Würzburg is a beautiful town in Bavaria, Germany, where I had the opportunity to spend my sabbatical with Dr Edgar Serfling in 1996. The university was a mecca for molecular immunology, and the scientists in this small institute were making major contributions to the understanding of basic immunology. Edgar, along with scientists Andris Avots, Stefan Klein-Hessling and Friederike Berberich-Siebelt, who have become good friends, were doing cutting-edge experiments to understand how IL-2 was secreted after a T cell recognized the antigen by the T cell receptors. Dr Hünig was studying the CD28 molecule and how it regulated signal two. His contributions have been critical to the discovery of key aspects of immune regulation.*

Prior to initiating the clinical trials, the drug was given to non-human primates to ensure that it was safe to give to humans. No major toxicity was observed, and all the studies done demonstrated that the drug was safe. After successful preclinical studies the European Medicines Agency (EMA) regulators approved the initiating of clinical trials.

The first human clinical trials were designed to give an extremely low dose of the drug, 0.1 mg/kg, 500 times lower than the dosage tested in the toxicology studies conducted using monkeys. Six healthy donors were given the drug at Northwick Park and St Mark's Hospital, London. The drug was given intravenously. Five minutes later, the participants complained of headache, pain, vomiting and fever and suffered catastrophic system organ failure. It was 13 March 2006. These major adverse events were not expected. All the men underwent a reaction called cytokine release syndrome (CRS). Their spleens were enlarged and the white blood cells disappeared from their blood. The hospital treated the patients, and by July, they were all discharged. But had they not been in a hospital setting, they would have surely died.

---

* Hünig, T. 'Manipulation of Regulatory T-cell Number and Function with CD28-specific Monoclonal Antibodies'. *Advances in Immunol.* 95, (2007): 111–48.

The drug was withdrawn from development in March 2006; the company TeGenero went bankrupt.*

What happened? A detailed investigation showed that the CRS caused by the drug was not due to contamination of the drug or incorrect dosing, but rather was a direct effect of the drug itself. The binding of the anti-CD28 to CD28 molecules on T cells, rather than blocking the delivery of signal two, resulted in super-activation, which resulted in a systemic hyperactivation of the immune system, since all T cells express CD28. Interestingly, animal testing of the drug had not predicted this major effect of the drug.

The UK-based regulatory agency that governed the oversight of the trial, the Medicines and Healthcare products Regulatory Agency (MHRA), provided a detailed report on the trial in May 2006. It found no deficiencies in TeGenero's animal studies, and all the records were in order, including all the dose measurements and administration processes. They concluded that the most likely cause of the reaction in the subjects was an unexpected biological effect in humans, which could not have been predicted in animal studies. The lesson learnt from this landmark failed study was the need to thoroughly evaluate the potential of hyperactivation of the immune system in various model systems prior to giving a drug to humans. Since 2006, no major unanticipated super-activation of the immune system has been reported.

---

* Attarawala, H. 'TGN1412: From Discovery to Disaster'. *J. Young Pharm.* 2 (2010): 332–6.

On the other side of the pond, in the US, Dr Carl June was also working on understanding the biology of CD28 molecules. If you remember, during the Cold War era in the early 1980s, Carl was sent to learn bone marrow transplantation techniques at Fred Hutch in Seattle. While there, he did extensive studies on the mechanisms of stimulation of T cells with a combination of signal one (CD3) and signal two (CD28) induced massive activation of T cells. He did significant research in understanding the complex biology of T cells. These experiments were seminal to the development of CAR-T cells.

The three E's of the immunology of cancer*

Tumours are notorious for creating an environment of suppressive factors that inhibit T cell activation. Dr June hypothesized that T cells that could be optimally activated outside the body and then reinjected should be able to kill tumours. Several researchers in the 1980s were making seminal findings that activation of the immune system indeed played an important role in the control of tumours. Dr Robert Schreiber, at the University of Missouri–St Louis, described the evolution of cancer in terms of three E's, namely, elimination, equilibrium and escape. All of us have some mutations occurring in some cells of our genome due

---

* Gavin, D.P., Old, L. and Schreiber, R. 'The Three Es of Cancer Immunoediting'. *Annual Reviews in Immunology* 22 (2004): 329–60.

to various insults such as radiation, pollutants, air quality, foods, etc. When there is a mutation, the protein product that is made by the gene looks foreign, and the immune system eliminates the tumour cell; this phenomenon is constantly occurring in our bodies, without our knowledge. This state is that of 'elimination'. Sometimes, however, the tumour starts to grow; first as a single cell, in a single organ or tissue. It is still very small, most of the time not diagnosed, and does not cause any overt symptoms. It is silent. This state is that of 'equilibrium'. In the final state, the tumour grows aggressively, spreads to different parts of the body (metastasis), secretes several immune-suppressive factors, creates blood vessels for itself to get nutrients (endostatins) and results in many major clinical symptoms. This phase is the state of 'escape'.

The stages of cancer are much like the four states of consciousness described in the Mandukya Upanishad, namely, waking, dreaming, deep sleep and the fourth state 'turiya', a state of absolute bliss, where one is realized. Similarly, the fourth state in cancer can be when the body is able to overcome the cancer through treatment. That cure is where innovation in the field of cancer immunotherapy is headed.

One of the ways to attack a tumour is to provide active T cells to the immune system. Israeli immunologists Zelig Eshhar and Gideon Gross devised an ingenious approach by expressing an antibody molecule on the T cell, called the CAR-T cells (for chimeric antigen receptor T cells).

Let's go back to our analogy of War to the immune system. After the terrorists have invaded the city, the general orders the air force (antibodies secreted by B cells which are like airborne target-specific missiles) and the army (the analogy of hand-to-hand combat, to cell-to-cell interaction mediated killing by cytotoxic T cells) to attack the terrorist. There is a 'special forces' team which comprises hand-to-hand combat soldiers, that can shoot missiles (a combination of the property of target-specific missiles [antibody] to the killing machinery of the field soldier [Cytotoxic T cell]).

Back to the CAR-T cells, Eshhar and Gross engineered the recognition domain of an antibody directed to an antigen expressed on a tumour cell (in this case CD19, which is expressed on the cell surface of B cell leukaemia).* This extracellular domain of the CAR recognizes CD19 positive tumour cells. The intracellular domain of the CAR was engineered with the signalling domains of the tail of CD3 and another molecule called 41BB. (Steven Rosenberg used a similar approach by using the cytoplasmic tail of CD28.) This approach empowered T cells from the cancer patient to be 'fitted' with a chimeric protein on its killer T cells that was easily able to recognize the cancer cell. Thus, when CAR-T cells were added to CD19-expressing tumour cells in the lab experiments, they successfully killed all the tumour cells.

---

* Credit for CAR also goes to Margo Roberts (Cell Genesys, Chimeric Receptor Molecules for Delivery of Co-Stimulatory Signals, US Patent 5,686,281, 11 November 1997) and Helene Finney (CellTech, Chimeric Receptors Providing Both Primary and Costimulatory Signaling in T Cells from a Single Gene Product. *Journal of Immunology*. 1998;161:2791–7).

Would this neat approach work in patients?

Carl June and Bruce Levine, working at the University of Pennsylvania, developed a process to translate the research work into a therapy for treatment of patients. Thus, when the CAR-T cells were administered to patients, these cells killed the CD19 positive leukaemic cells, and cured the cancer of many patients. This treatment has resulted in a paradigm shift in the treatment of patients with cancer.

In parallel, Dr James Allison, had performed a very interesting experiment while studying a molecule, called CTLA4, which also bound to CD80 and CD86 molecules on APC, with higher affinity. Interestingly, when he injected mice that had tumours with an anti-CTLA4 antibody, the tumours vanished.

Jim Allison is white-bearded scientist, who has been doing work in the area of basic immunology all his life. Born in Alice, Texas, he did his early work in the University of Texas, and then moved to the University of California at Berkeley, where he did his seminal work in discovery of the role of CTLA4 in termination of the immune response. He won the Nobel Prize for this work along with Tasuku Honjo, from Kyoto University, Japan. The persistence of Dr Allison in bringing the discovery he had made in the laboratory to treating patients with cancer, a story of bench-to-bedside, is told in the documentary *Breakthrough*.

To understand the amazing discovery made by Dr Allison, we need to go back to the analogy of the terrorist versus armed forces battle. In our story, the armed forces destroy the terrorist and his gang. Now the city is filled with armed personnel. These forces have to go back to their base and vacate the city. The instructions to leave and return to base after the job is done are also given by the general.

What Dr Allison discovered is that tumour cells (i.e., the terrorist in our analogy) cleverly send the return-to-base signal right at the beginning of the fight, when they invade the 'city'. Thus, the armed forces never receive the orders to come to battle. The tumour cells do this by tricking the immune system to receive the termination signal prematurely. As a result, T cells in our body do not kill the tumour cells. This is the mechanism of escape in the three-E process of tumour immunology. Dr Allison discovered that blocking this termination signal delivered by the tumour cells activates T cells, which in turn kill the tumour and cure the patient.

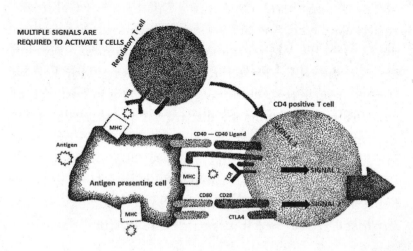

The figure above with multiple signals, shows the technical details for the advanced reader. The molecule that is upregulated by tumour cells is CTLA4 on T cells. Binding of CTLA4 to CD80 and CD86 delivers a stop signal to T cells, instructing them to terminate the immune response. In normal cells (for example, when the immune response is activated to fight bacteria or viruses), CTLA4 is expressed by T cells at a late stage of the immune response, after the pathogens have been eliminated. CTLA4 is upregulated to shut off the immune system, after the battle has been won. In the case of several tumours, the tumours cleverly secrete factors that force the upregulation of CTLA4 on T cells prematurely, preventing the activation of T cells in the first place. This mistimed upregulation of CTLA4 is the mechanism by which tumours escape being killed.

In the animal experiment that Dr Allison conducted, mice with tumours were treated with an anti-CTLA4 antibody, which blocked the binding of CTLA4 to CD80 and CD86 on APC. The anti-CTLA4 antibody induced activation of the T cells in the mice, which then killed the tumour and cured the mice. Tasuku Honjo, from Kyoto University, a physician-scientist, made a similar discovery with another pair of molecules, the programmed death receptor (PD-1) and the molecule it interacts with, programmed death receptor ligand (PD-1L). PD-1 is generally expressed on T cells, and when it binds to PD-1L, it shuts down the T cell activation. Blocking the PD-1 and PD-1L interaction enhances the ability of the immune system to kill tumours.

The anti-CTLA4 antibody was developed by Bristol Myers Squibb (BMS) as ipilimumab (short name ipi, and brand name Yervoy), and the anti-PD1 antibody was developed by Merck as pembrolizumab (short name pembro, and brand name Keytruda). Good friends of mine who have worked on Keytruda are Gargi Maheshwari, a chemical engineer from New Delhi who did her PhD from Caltech and MIT and headed the manufacturing of Keytruda; and Prashant Nikam, who did his PhD from Ohio State in health economics and MBA from the Wharton School of Business and heads one of the marketing groups for Keytruda. They have fascinating stories on the remarkable effects of this revolutionary drug in curing certain patients with cancer. Working on the development of this molecule has been an inflection point in their careers. Both drugs, ipi and pembro, are being used to treat patients with various types of cancer. But this is just the beginning, since only 10 to 30 per cent of patients are 'cured', that is, they have a survival rate of greater than five years. A deeper understanding of the cells and molecules of the immune system will enable greater efficacy.[*]

---

[*] Anderson, W. 'The Checkpoint Immunotherapy Revolution: What Started as a Trickle Has Become a Flood, Despite Some Daunting Adverse Effects; New Drugs, Indications, and Combinations Continue to Emerge'. *Pharmacy and Therapeutics* 41 (2016): 185–91.

One major social aspect of this miraculous revolutionary treatment is the cost. Currently, it costs between $1,00,000 and $5,00,000 per year per patient. It has been estimated that the cost to society for treatment of the few cancer patients is more than $2 billion per year. There are many factors associated with the cost of drugs. Manufacturing this specialized class of biological drugs requires extremely sophisticated facilities. The clinical trials to test them to ensure safety and efficacy are also very expensive. The overall costs to a company of each of these drugs is now $1 billion (approximately Rs 7000 crore). The distribution and access to patients in various parts of the world are also major challenges in the supply chain. Thus, manufacturing these life-saving drugs and enabling affordable treatment is one of the holy grails of cancer immunotherapy. This topic is so important that it needs another book by health economists and public health officials. Several references are provided for the interested reader to explore this topic further.

5

The Story of Cell Therapy

Engineering cells to become killers.

I could have started this chapter with a story about how treatment of a patient with stem cells resulted in a miraculous cure. But then, I could also have told an equally sensational story about a stem cell treatment gone bad. Stem cells are a central topic of popular science, and any and every advance in the field makes sensational news in media and social media.

To explain the complex and fascinating biology of stem cells, let us use the analogy of society. After birth, a baby stays at home for about three years. Then, we all go to elementary school, middle school, high school and college. During the education process we learn right from wrong, among many other things. After graduation, each person performs a different job in society. Doctors, construction workers, engineers, scientists, painters, jugglers, performing artists, etc. Each role is critical in maintaining harmony in society. Stem cells are the baby that grows up and differentiates into different types of cells, which make the various organ systems of our body.

In the development of stem cells, after the sperm fertilizes the ovum, there is an organized, systematic doubling of these cells, called clones of the stem cells. At this stage these are christened 'totipotent' stem cells. The clones grow by doubling, from two to four, to eight, to sixteen, to thirty-two, and so on. The DNA in each cell is instructed to differentiate into a daughter cell that performs activities that are different from the parent. These pluripotent stem cells can develop a few, but not all organs (follow the branch of a tree in the figure below; starting at the stem cell, and then differentiating into various cells which make up different organs). There is then further differentiation, and these stem cells are committed to specific systems or organs, such as muscles, the immune system, neurons, liver cells, etc. It is a unidirectional differentiation, i.e. a stem cell differentiated into a cell of an organ, and not in the reverse direction. Right? Wrong.

While majority of the stem cells terminally differentiate into their respective organs, there are stem cells in adults that are multipotent, i.e., they can differentiate into various cell types and in turn, organs. These cells are abundant in cord blood. Researchers Shinya Yamanaka, a senior investigator at Gladstone Institute in San Francisco, and John Gurdon, founder of the Gurdon Institute at

STEM CELLS

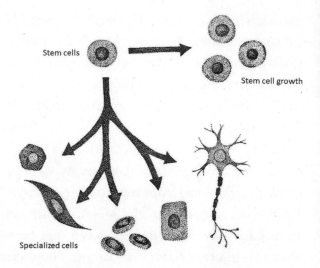

Stem cells

Stem cell growth

Specialized cells

Cambridge, UK, studied the differentiation of stem cells and discovered the key genes that are required for stem cells to differentiate from totipotent and pluripotent to multipotent stem cells.*

Totipotent stem cells are the earliest cells formed after the fertilization of the egg by the sperm and can give rise to all other cell types, such as liver, lung, heart, etc. Pluripotent cells are the next step of differentiation and can develop into some but not all organs. And finally, multipotent stem cells can develop into any of a family of related cells, for example, blood multipotent cells can develop into all the cell types of blood.

---

* Collman, A. 'Profile of John Gurdon and Shinya Yamanaka, 2012 Nobel Laureates in Medicine or Physiology'. *Proceedings of the National Academy of Sciences (USA)*. 110 (2013): 5740–41.

Shinya Yamanaka and John Gurdon's discovery showed the process that could change these cell-fates at will by introducing specific genes. These genes are termed 'Yamanaka transcription factors'. Adding these four specific genes to any cell coerces it to de-differentiate into a pluripotent stem cell, and hence it is termed an 'inducible pluripotent stem cell' (iPSC). An iPSC can then be differentiated into specific cell types and used as a 'source' of stem cells for treating that organ. Shinya Yamanaka and John B. Gurdon were awarded the Nobel Prize in Physiology or Medicine in 2012 'for the discovery that mature cells can be reprogrammed to become pluripotent', i.e., mature cells can be converted into stem cells.

Every human being has around 30,000 genes. In fact, we have two copies of each of those genes, one inherited from our mother, the other from our father. Our genome is extremely complex, and even after twenty years of human genome sequencing, we have only understood a small fraction of the functions of genes. Astonishingly, of the approximately 30,000 genes that are expressed by humans, only about 754 genes for proteins have been targets for therapies.* A huge amount of work needs to be done before we start using stem cells to treat diseases. The groups that are addressing this formidable challenge are hampered by negative outcomes and are learning from

---

* Hopkins, A.L. and Groom, C.R. 'The Druggable Genome'. *Nature Reviews Drug Discovery* 1 (2002): 727–30.

them as they persist in changing the paradigm of treatment of human disease.

Let us return to the analogy of society to understand the genesis of the immune system. After completing high school, a person enters university. A bachelor's degree in science comprises general subjects such as zoology, botany, chemistry, physics and statistics. A degree in the arts comprises classes in history, geography, philosophy, sociology, literature, etc., and a degree in commerce comprises economics, accounting, taxation, audit, business management, etc. Thus, those who earn a bachelor's degree are generalists, capable of 'differentiating' into any specialty. To specialize, one requires the advanced training of graduate school, a master's or a PhD. The decision to choose a particular subject is based on innumerable factors such as aptitude, environmental factors, social and genetic background.

Like the person who has been trained for a particular job in society, the precursor cell that is committed to developing the immune system learns and differentiates into three branches: a precursor for red blood cells, white blood cells and platelet cells. Let us follow the white blood cell precursor along the branched tree.

Some of these cells leave their birthplace, the bone marrow, and travel to the thymus (the college of the immune system). These cells are T-cell precursors, so named for their college the 'T'hymus. Here, the stem cells committed to becoming T cells of the immune system are 'educated' on how to differentiate self-antigens and non-self (foreign)

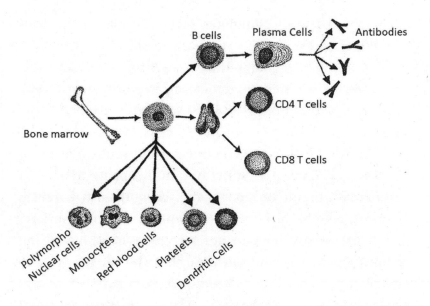

antigens. All the cells that enter the thymus for education are programmed to die unless they receive an appropriate signal that protects them from this death. Death of cells is the 'norm'. Unless these cells are recused by stimulatory signals given by adjacent cells, they die (hence the term: programmed to die). These T cell precursors express two proteins, which are termed as T cell receptors (TCR). The TCRs have specific binding regions (called complementarity determining regions [CDR]) that recognize self and foreign antigens and trigger biochemical signals to activate them. These biochemical signals comprise enzymatic reactions that occur in a cascade of events, hence called 'signals' (similar to electrical signal transmitted through a wire). In the thymus, a strong recognition signal (of high affinity) sends a signal and eliminates them. The recognition of an antigen in the thymus (typically a SELF antigen) by a T cell is a trigger (signal) to kill; since if this T cell survives, and enters the systemic circulation, it will recognize self antigens in the body, and cause autoimmunity. This period of training to equip the T cells to recognize self-antigens (and be killed) is a critical event in the education process (called negative selection). In this phase, the T cell precursors capable of recognizing self-antigens (therefore harmful) need to be eliminated to prevent autoimmunity. T cell precursors that do not recognize anything in the thymus are useless and die since they do not receive any signal to protect them from programmed cell death. Only those T cells that receive a weak recognition signal (through the TCR) are protected from programmed cell death (positive selection) and graduate to become mature T cells. About 98 per cent of the T cell precursors that go through the thymic education process of positive and negative selection die; only 2 per cent mature. The process of ensuring the elimination of the cells is very robust. The mature cells then move out of the thymus and into the peripheral organs (such as the spleen and lymph nodes) and blood and are critical for protecting the immune system from invading foreign antigens.

Another branch of stem cells committed to the immune system remains in the bone marrow and differentiates into B cells. These cells develop the receptor for recognition of antigens, called the immunoglobulins or antibodies.

Selection in the Thymus

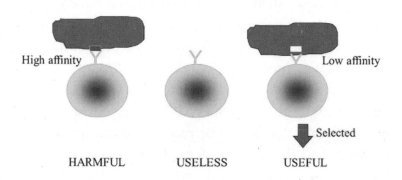

Immunoglobulins expressed on the membrane of B cells are called B cell receptors (BCRs); while those that are secreted are called antibodies. BCRs also undergo an education process similar to that for T cells (negative and positive selection), mature and graduate to transfer to the peripheral organs (spleen) and blood.

The field of immunology is extremely young, in relative terms. While the basic concepts of mathematics were defined hundreds, if not thousands, of years ago, and the laws of physics a few hundred years ago, the major basic concepts of immunology began to be discovered only in the 1960s. In this respect, Max Cooper (Emory University School of Medicine, Atlanta, California and Jacques Miller (Walter and Eliza Hall Institute Medical Research, Australia), were awarded the Lasker Award (the US equivalent of the Nobel Prize) in 2019 for their seminal discoveries on T and B cells.

The birth of bone marrow transplantation

Bone marrow stem cell transplantation (BMT) was pioneered by American physicians E. Donnall Thomas, from Cooperstown, New York, in identical twins. He developed the process for BMT in genetically identical donors. Robert A. Good initiated the process in non-identical twins at the Memorial Sloan Kettering Institute in New York, that does not require genetically identical donors. I had the fortune of working with Robert Good when I was doing my post-doctoral fellowship with Savita Pahwa at North Shore University Hospital in New York. He was a well-built man with a commanding presence. He has done seminal work in the field and is considered to be the father of modern immunology. Both these processes of BMT, revolutionary in their own way, have transformed the treatment of several lethal diseases, including leukaemia. The BMT process requires donors who are matched with the recipients through several genetic tests. Since 1968, after the first BMT, hundreds of severe combined immunodeficiency (SCID) patients have been treated, nay, cured. The success rate is an amazing 80 per cent or so when a matched donor is available. The rate of cure has dramatically increased due to post-transplant management of infectious diseases and a good nutritional regimen. The widespread use of BMT with mismatched donors has had limited success, due to graft-versus-host disease reactions, advanced age of the recipient, which results in higher infection rates and lack of long-term stability, resulting in elimination of the graft, of the transplanted cells.

Siddhartha Mukherjee has elegantly written about the story of BMT in the *New Yorker*.* He states, 'New living drugs made from patients' own cells can cure once incurable cancers—but can we afford them?' BMT is such a standard procedure in the arsenal of medical treatments that it is taught to fourth grade children.† The reader is urged to read some of these articles and books for a deeper understanding of this technology, which has revolutionized the treatment of deadly diseases. This learning has not come easy, and the field went through many inflection points.

BMT requires a donor. *Can the donor be the patient themselves?* This question was asked by the pioneers in this type of gene therapy, William French Anderson and Michael Blaese. These clinical scientists understood both molecular biology and the clinical aspects of diseases. They were pioneers in converting ideas in the laboratory to treatment of patients, a field called translational science.

On 14 September 1990, Ashanti DeSilva was the first patient treated with gene therapy under the direction of Drs French Anderson and Blaese at the National Institutes of Health in Bethesda. Ashanti was about four years old. She was dying because she had no immune system.

---

* Mukherjee, S. 'The Promise and Price of Cellular Therapies'. *New Yorker*, 15 July 2019.
† Baby Professor. 'The Bone Marrow Transplant'—Biology 4th Grade | Children's Biology Books. Speedy Publishing LLC. (2017).

Her parents Raj and Van DeSilva were desperate. The disease she had was a rare immune disorder caused by the mutation of a gene for an enzyme adenosine deaminase (ADA) on both her chromosomes, in the cells of the bone marrow. ADA is an enzyme that is required for differentiation of a stem cell into T cells. It plays a crucial role in our resistance to disease. Without it, special white blood cells called T cells die off. Without T cells, ADA-deficient children are wide open to the attacks of viruses and bacteria. Typically, we have two copies of the gene (one on each chromosome from our parents). Both genes were mutated; if either was not, she would have been healthy.

As noted above in the analogy of society, these stem cells of the bone marrow are the source for the formation of the entire immune system. Due to this mutation, the bone marrow cells of these patients do not have the ability to differentiate into T cells and B cells, and therefore the immune system does not develop. This condition results in severe (combined) immune deficiency. Combined, because patients lack both T and B cells. The disease occurs in one in 50,000 to one in 1,00,000 live births, in different parts of the world.

Since Ashanti did not have a suitable genetically matched donor, Drs French Anderson and Blaese isolated the immune stem cells from her own bone marrow. They then inserted the ADA gene into her stem cells. For this purpose, they engineered the genes of a virus (retrovirus) with the normal ADA gene. Her stem cells were then infected with this engineered virus so that the cells now had the normal ADA gene. These engineered cells were transplanted into Ashanti. Astonishingly, the treatment was a success. Her immune system developed. She went back to school and is now a young woman pursuing a normal life. The achievement of this trial was the beginning of the field of gene therapy. But not all trials had such success stories.

The field of gene therapy came under siege in the early 2000s. The death of Jesse Gelsinger (in 1999) was a devastating event that made scientists, regulators and even patients wary of trying something new. (Note: we shall review this story of Jesse Gelsinger in the next chapter on Gene Therapy.) French researchers Alain Fischer and Marina Cavazzana-Calvo embarked on a bold new study to treat patients with SCID. They used a modified virus by introducing the gene for ADA in the viral genome. This process is called a viral vector which transports the gene into the cell. The viral vector transports the gene into the cell, enables expression of the ADA protein, and results in treatment of SCID patients (sometimes called Bubble Boy disease).

In this form of SCID, children are born with another mutation of a gene. This disease occurs due to lack of a critical receptor on the bone marrow stem cell, called the interleukin 2 receptor γ, which is a receptor required for T cell growth. This defect results in children being vulnerable to infections and dying from them. In 1976, this disease was depicted in the movie *The Boy in the Plastic Bubble* starring John Travolta in the titular role. There were very few treatment options for this disease, and BMT with a genetically identical donor (usually sibling or parent) was the standard of care. It had a low probability of success.

Studying the potential of gene therapy for the treatment of patients with this disease had very strong justification. Animal studies had proven that the therapy could help fix the mutation of the interleukin 2 receptor gamma chain (IL2Rγ) gene. Extensive toxicology studies were performed to ensure the treatment had minimal side effects.[*] The procedure was less intrusive than adenovirus vectors since these retroviral vectors were not injected directly into the patient. In this case, the retroviral vector expressing the IL2Rγ gene was used to infect stem cells only in tissue culture flasks and not in the body.

To enable the process of inserting the normal gene, bone marrow stem cells from the patient were grown and expanded in a flask in the laboratory. The viral vector was added to the cells in the flask, where it entered the bone marrow cells. The cells, now carrying the normal IL2Rγ gene, were washed extensively of the free virus, to remove any free virus, and injected back into the patient. There was no free virus injected into the patients. Thus, the belief was that this procedure should not result in any side effects, like those seen in the case of Jesse Gelsinger.

---

[*] Fischer, A. and Hacein-Bey-Abina, S. 'Gene Therapy for Severe Combined Immunodeficiencies and Beyond'. *Journal of Experimental Medicine* 217 (2019): e20190607.

The bone marrow stem cells transduced with the retrovirus expressing the normal version of the defective gene were now expressing the normal IL2Rγ gene and were able to grow in the SCID patient's body and form normal T and B cells. The patient was cured! It was a miraculous treatment. There was celebration in the gene therapy community, especially after a low in the field following Jesse Gelsinger's death.

But alas, another disastrous event awaited the field of gene therapy.

The children who had been treated with the virus vector expressing the normal IL2Rγ gene started developing symptoms of leukaemia. The T cells in their body started to grow uncontrollably. Cancer. The deadliest diagnosis for any individual, let alone someone who has been cured of another lethal disease.

Questions were asked. i) How did this happen? ii) Was the scientific mechanism of the insertional mutation understood? iii) Could these cancers have been anticipated? iv) What could be done to ensure situations like this would not happen again? v) Were there consequences to these induced cancers? vi) Why was there a lack of understanding of the biology of the disease and the process of treatment? vii) What were the societal implications of the results of such clinical studies?

Intensive investigations began. Molecular biologists got back to work to understand why the cells began to grow uncontrollably. In normal healthy individuals,

IL-2 is secreted by T cells themselves and binds to the IL2R (IL-2 receptor). This binding event stimulates the growth of T cells. Normally, once the T cells have done their job (of killing the infected cells), IL-2 secretion is stopped and the T cells stop growing.

In the case of a SCID patient treated with the transduced IL2Rγ-expressing stem cell, IL-2 was not required for the cells to grow. The cells started growing by themselves. They had a mind of their own. What had happened was that the gene for IL2Rγ was inserted randomly into the chromosome of the cells at a location where it could instruct the cell to grow without the need for IL-2. Like a villain in a James Bond movie, it 'wanted to take over the world'.

The scientists in the field did not give up. In the investigation that ensued, it was discovered that the DNA used in the retrovirus vector with the IL2Rγ insertion had sequences that promoted insertion into the site where it transformed the normal cell into a cancer cell. These sequences were deleted in the next version of the retrovirus vector, and an additional sequence that made the vector self-inactivating (SIN) was added. This molecular engineering of the viral vector made the vector safe(r).

Nine boys were treated with the new self-inactivating vector, of which seven restored their immune responses without causing leukaemia. At the time of writing, it was still too early to claim success. The treatment times range from sixteen to forty-three months. Because leukaemia takes a long time to develop, the boys will be followed for at least fifteen years before success is claimed.

Gene therapy is an extremely difficult nut to crack. It is after all the holy grail of medicine. Progress reports are often presented at scientific and medical meetings, and if the media attends, articles follow. That is why the headlines and endless repetition of press releases via aggregators following publication in a major journal can seem like echoes. They are.

Scientific proof that gene therapy works effectively in the long term, doesn't exist. Every result sparks new questions and no conclusion is ever final, for what we learn continually teaches us how much more we need to know. If science ever had the final word on something, we would still think the Earth is flat, that proteins are the genetic material, and that the entire human genome encodes protein.

Dr Donald Kohn, from University of California at Los Angeles, CA, elegantly summed up the significance of the SCID gene therapy trial results: 'It's a reflection of the iterative bench-to-bedside process, with initial clinical observations spurring further research studies and a next generation of treatments brought to the clinic. For this specific disease, SCID-X1, this study represents a do-over in using the indisputable logic of gene therapy to treat this most responsive disorder, using prior lessons to do it even better.'

Dr James M. Wilson, from the University of Pennsylvania, said: 'Gene therapy is a classic disruptive technology. It's so different, and it will impact the entire practice of medicine. But we as a society will figure it out. We'll have some successes, we'll have some failures. It's still science, we're still learning, this is not routine. We're at the very beginning.'

Twenty years after the first gene-modified bone marrow transplants were done, the procedures to do such therapies have become standard practice. The vectors are far better designed. Self-inactivating regulatory genes are now inserted into the vectors. The SIN ensures that if something goes wrong in the treatment, there is a way out. The field of gene-modified BMT is here to stay. While a lot has been achieved, there is much more to be done to further refine the system.

As an outcome of the efforts to improve BMT therapy, another cell therapy, chimeric antigen receptor T cells (CAR-T cell), has emerged.

The year was about 1999. Carl June and Bruce Levine had just moved from the Naval Medical Center in Washington, D.C. to the University of Pennsylvania. I had been following their work on how T cells in HIV infection were significantly compromised and how signals transmitted through a costimulatory molecule on T cells made them resistant to HIV infection. A very interesting observation that even today requires some understanding. I was working in the department of medical genetics in the Institute for Human Gene Therapy with Jim Wilson. My labs and office were adjacent to Carl and Bruce's labs.

We shared our experiences and experimental results in journal clubs, meetings in the cafeteria and corridor conversations. I continue to discuss immunology with Bruce and Carl to this day. In fact, I am now teaching courses on regulatory aspects of drug development at the University of Pennsylvania. This rich environment of highly qualified research scientists sharing ideas every day is one of the most important elements of innovative discoveries.

Carl and Bruce had been working together for many years. Carl is the clinician, and Bruce the scientist. Both were passionate about getting CAR-T cells to the clinic. They started working on a process to grow human T cells so that they could be manipulated in the lab and potentially reinfused into patients. They were hoping to expand them exponentially. Carl had been trained in BMT processes with E. Donnall Thomas. He had studied the signalling mechanisms of CD28 molecules that enabled T cells to grow (these are the inflection points in his career), and he was in the right place at the right time—the University of Pennsylvania, the heart of gene therapy in the late 1990s. Malcolm Gladwell would call this phenomenon of 'coupling' two independent events in his book *Talking to Strangers*. All these experiences of Carl and Bruce enabled them to develop a process for genetically engineering a chimeric antigen receptor into T cells and unleashing them to kill tumour cells when injected in vivo, i.e., injected into the body of the patient. The process of using CAR-T cells to 'cure' certain types of leukaemia was developed by many key scientists working across cities. Collaboration was key to the success. The story of CAR-T cells below, told by many, is my version based on my personal experience of observing Carl and Bruce.

'The overnight success of CAR-T cells in curing some kinds of leukaemia has taken more than twenty years,' Bruce Levine often says at the opening of talks he is invited to give on the subject. When Carl and Bruce came with their team in 1996 to UPenn, they had started growing T cells in vitro*, i.e., in flasks in the laboratory, by stimulating them with a combination of antibodies to CD3 and CD28 (receptors on T cells that deliver signal one and signal two). T cells responded by proliferating by up to 500-fold. The process to grow these cells requires a sterile environment where no other infections can contaminate the cells. When Jim Wilson's gene therapy clinical programme for adenovirus vectors was being shut down due to the tragedy of Jesse Gelsinger, a ready-made good manufacturing practice (GMP) facility was now available to grow the T cells: the Maloney building at the Hospital of the University of Pennsylvania. I had been to this facility several times when adenovirus vectors were being made there. It is very clean. Just how clean is defined by the International Standards Organization

---

* June, Carl. 'A "Living Drug" That Could Change the Way We Treat Cancer'. *TEDMED*, Nov. 2018.

(ISO)*, which defines air quality that ranges from ISO-9 (room air) to ISO-1 (no more than two particles of greater than 2 microns [dust size] per metre square) to ensure prevention of infections. The Maloney GMP facility was ranked at ISO-4 (no more than 10,000 particles of greater than 5 microns per metre square), which is as clean as an operating theatre. The scientists who work in this facility gown up from head to toe and work in a closed system, where airflow is prevented from external air interactions by air filters.

The CAR itself is a very clever tool, first designed by Israeli immunologist Zelig Eshhar of the Weissman Institute in Israel, working with Steven Rosenberg at National Institutes of Health. He took the ability of the antigen-binding domain of an antibody molecule (directed against a tumour antigen, CD19) and fused it to a cytoplasmic domain of the T cell receptor signalling tail, CD3-zeta (CD3ζ). This designer molecule does not exist in nature. It is a chimera. In Hindu mythology, Narasimha, Lord Krishna's half-lion and half-human avatar, was born to kill the demon Narakasura. CAR is the same thing. A chimeric molecule developed to kill the demon, leukaemic cells.

How does one insert a CAR into a T cell? There were many folks who were working on developing processes to insert genes into cells during the 1990s. Carl and Bruce were also working on HIV to develop a vector system to

---

* https://en.wikipedia.org/wiki/Cleanroom

CAR-T CELLS

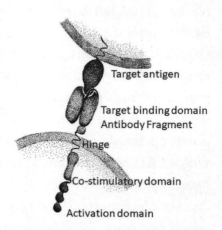

infect non-dividing cells. This vector comes from the same family of viruses as HIV and lentivirus. Inder Verma and Luigi Naldini working at the Salk Institute had developed an elegant process to use the 'good' aspects of HIV (namely its ability to infect and transport DNA to the nucleus) and remove its negative aspect (causing immune deficiency). This virus when manipulated is a vector whose sole function is to transport DNA into specific cells.

The CAR protein was made by fusing the DNA expressing the gene for the antigen-binding region of the anti-CD19 and the cytoplasmic tail of the CD3ζ. This chimeric DNA was inserted into a lentivirus. This lentivirus vector expressing the CAR was used to infect T cells. The T cells (isolated from a patient with B cell leukaemia, which expresses the CD19 protein) were expanded by stimulating (and thereby activating them to proliferate) them with anti-CD3+anti-CD28 antibodies which stimulate T cells through the CD3 and CD28 molecules. Infection of these cells with the CAR-containing lentivirus induces the expression of the anti-CD19 antibody on their surfaces. The outer portion, the antibody-portion of the chimera, of the CAR is able to recognize CD19 positive leukaemic tumour cells. The bottom portion of the CAR consists of the cytoplasmic tail of CD3 molecules, which enables transmission of the biochemical signal to the T cell, which then activates the 'killing machinery'. This machinery is made of proteins called perforins (which make pores in target cells) and granzymes (which are extremely potent proteolytic enzymes that digest other proteins). Upon binding of the CD19-CAR to CD19 tumour, the killer signal is transmitted and perforins and granzymes do the rest, killing the leukaemic cells. Precisely. Accurately. Without inflammatory responses. The tumour is dissolved and cancer is cured. An amazing discovery.

CAR-T cell therapy has revolutionized the treatment of leukaemia and various types of cancers. The scientific basis of CAR-T cells has been established through research conducted over the past two decades, as well as by the recent regulatory approvals of these therapies for the treatment of acute lymphocytic leukaemia and other tumour types. The process of development of CAR-T cell therapy requires a personalized medicine approach. A patient's lymphocytes are transfected with lentiviral vectors expressing chimeric receptors. These cells are grown in Good Manufacturing Process (GMP) suites closely associated with hospital-based infrastructure. The process of treatment of patients with leukaemia is described in a workflow as 'vein-to-vein'. A patient's lymphocytes are isolated from blood drawn from the vein, stably transfected with the chimeric receptor, and introduced back to the patient through an intravenous injection. The process requires twenty-one days.

The clinical trials for approval of the therapy were long and arduous. The first CAR-T cell therapy was approved by the FDA on 30 August 2017. It was called Kymriah (pronounced kim-rye-ah) and was the result of a collaboration between scientists at the University of Pennsylvania and the giant pharmaceutical company Novartis. It took more than ten years and hundreds of scientists, administrators, clinicians, nurses' regulators, and many other teams to develop the process, submit the application and approve the therapy, which has a definitive benefit with manageable side effects. Another advisory committee (Ad-Comm). The Ad-Comm is initiated by the US FDA where they invite experts in the field to review the scientific data submitted for approval, and provide a recommendation for approval. This process is completely transparent to the public. The details of which are published by the FDA*. The sessions are broadcast live on the web around the world.

---

* BLA 125646. Tisagenlecleucel. FDA Briefing Book (2017). https://www.fda.gov/media/106081/download

The review of the results of the Ad-Comm was broadcast on live TV. The advisory committee voted unanimously ten to zero in favour of the benefit-risk profile of this novel therapy. The product is a 'living drug' since it comprises the living cells of the patient, which are transformed to become cancer-killing cells. The efficacy of the treatment of adult and child patients with a specific kind of blood cancer, called B cell acute lymphoblastic leukaemia (B-ALL) is higher than 83 per cent, as measured by a response to therapy, and greater than 40 per cent of them have survived for more than a year. Emily Whitehead, the poster child for receiving this treatment, has survived for more than nine years and is doing extremely well. This treatment was almost a miracle, since these patients would otherwise have died within a few months given the advanced stage of their cancer.

In the past few years, four new CAR-T cell therapies have been approved and several hundred are being developed around the world. This therapy has revolutionized the treatment of some kinds of cancers. Neil Canavan has written elegantly about the scientists who have made a major contribution to CAR-T cell therapy in his book *The Cure Within.** Hundreds of companies and academic institutions are collaborating to develop these gene-modified cell therapies using novel targets, different cell

---

* Canavan, N. *A Cure Within: Scientists Unleashing the Immune System to Kill Cancer.* (New York: Cold Spring Harbor Press, 2017).

types and manufacturing processes. The individualized, custom-made autologous CAR-T cell production process platform remains a significant limiting factor for its large-scale clinical application. In this respect, the advances in standardization and automation of the process can significantly reduce costs. Innovation in the development of off-the-shelf, ready-to-use universal killer cells can enable scale-up. While this cell therapy is widely used in the US, Europe and China, there is very limited development of it in developing countries in Asia, Africa and Latin America. From an Indian perspective, there are many challenges such as manufacturing requirements, operational logistics and regulatory processes that need to be considered to ensure high-quality gene-modified cell therapies. A lot of work needs to be done to overcome the challenges to affordability and scalability.

Three companies in India have started working on CAR-T cell therapies. ImmunoACT (a collaboration of IIT-Bombay and Tata Memorial Hospital) in Mumbai, Immuneel Therapeutics in Bangalore, and Intas in Ahmedabad. This is just the beginning of making CAR-T cell therapy more accessible in India.

6

The Story of Gene Therapy

Trials and tribulations in the
complicated path of gene therapy.

The process of drug development involves a systematic characterization of the drug, as well as a deep understanding of the pathogenesis of the disease and the mechanism by which the drug acts on the disease. At the University of Pennsylvania, Drs James Wilson and Mark Batshaw were embarking on the treatment of a rare genetic disease, ornithine transcarbamylase (OTC) deficiency. OTC is a disease in which patients have a mutation in the gene for this enzyme. OTC deficiency results in the absence of this enzyme in the pathway by which the protein we consume is converted to urea and either used by the body to create energy or excreted through urine. We don't think twice about eating protein in our foods. However, someone with OTC deficiency cannot convert protein into energy or urea because of the absence of the enzyme OTC. The cascade of events that occurs in the body after protein is consumed results in the formation of an intermediate chemical called ammonia. Ammonia travels to the brain of the patient and can cause damage, which results in inflammation in the brain. This is bad news for the body, and the patient finally dies of severe brain damage. The symptoms can include seizures, diminished muscle tone, decreased liver function and respiratory abnormalities. It is a lethal disease, with no cure.

Using gene therapy to cure this disease was considered possible because it is caused by the mutation of a single gene. The thinking in the field was clear: correct the single gene defect in the liver, and the disease would be cured.

We have already discussed what a gene is in Chapter 1. It is made up of a chemical substance called nucleotide. There are four nucleotides: A(denine), C(ytosine), T(hymine) and G(uanine). These nucleotides, in various permutations and combinations, spell out our entire genome. A mutation in any of these nucleotides causes some dysfunction of the gene and results in a disease.

Let me explain this through an analogy.

In my sister Anjali Rao's house, there is a tradition of the entire family participating in the process of making meals. Anjali's day starts at 5 a.m. She is a busy physician and gets up early in the morning to plan the meals for the entire family. She writes down the menu for the day in a register. Okra, chana, arbi, dal, raita, roti, papad and kheer.

The process for making each item on the menu is written in the recipe book that our mother had written from notes from her mother. Anjali then keeps the register on the dining table. At about 8 a.m., Uncle Rao (her father-in-law) reads the menu for the day noted in the register. Next, he looks up the recipes for the dishes on the menu and gathers all the ingredients required for each, including the special family masala, and lays everything out neatly in the kitchen. At 11 a.m., the cook, Venkatamma, arrives. She cuts all the vegetables as instructed by the recipe, adds the masala and cooks the dishes. She places the dishes in a Styrofoam box. At 8 p.m., the Rao household opens the Styrofoam box and consumes the delicious, hot dinner. The process is efficient. Most of the time each person involved in the process does not even see the next person in the 'assembly line', yet all the messages are transmitted seamlessly. This process has been going on without any major failures for the past forty years.

Did you get the analogy of the recipe book (DNA) to the ingredients of the recipe (RNA), to making the food (protein)?

The recipe book is the DNA sequence of the gene in the genome. The recipe book was written by Anjali's mother and transmitted to her daughter. Writing the menu for the day is equivalent to the regulation of the DNA: which proteins need to be expressed (on each day, in each cell, in each organ, etc.). Reading the menu is akin to transcription of DNA (the recipe) to the messenger RNA (ingredients). Cutting the vegetables and preparing the masala is like processing the messenger

RNA and transferring to the ribosome (kitchen). Cooking the ingredients to convert them into edible food is the equivalent of conversion of functional proteins. The spices are the post-translational modifications that are required for the protein to function (for the food to be tasty). And eating the dinner is the source of energy for the cells, organs and body.

In order to explain the complex science of treatment of patients with genetic diseases with genes, it was important to understand the analogy of recipe-to-food. In the case of the rare disease called Ornithine Transcarbamylase (OTC) deficiency, the gene (DNA sequence) for this enzyme (the recipe) is defective; hence the conversion of the DNA to RNA (ingredients) is wrong, hence the protein (the food) made is defective. The lack of OTC enzyme in patients it results in severe brain damage and death, early in life. The reason for this disease biology is that OTC enzyme is required for the protein in food to be converted to urea (i.e. metabolism of the protein), which is then excreted. In patients with OTC deficiency, the protein in the food that they consume is not converted successfully to urea, instead it results in an intermediate metabolite, called ammonia. This ammonia is extremely toxic to brain cells, hence when children with this disease consume proteins, their brain gets damaged. The hypothesis for the gene therapy for OTC deficiency, is expression of the normal OTC gene in patients, will correct the genetic defect.

Mark Batshaw specializes in studying and treating patients with diseases that affect the functions of the liver and is the leading expert in treatment of patients with OTC deficiency. Only one in 80,000 people are affected by the mutation that causes this rare disease. Identifying patients with such a rare disease is like looking for a needle in a haystack.

James (Jim) M. Wilson is an extraordinarily gifted physician scientist. He did his MD and then his PhD with Phillip Sharp, a Nobel laureate. Phillip Sharp has discovered how many genes make one protein by a phenomenon called gene splicing (Uncle Rao's job in the analogy above). Jim then worked with Francis Collins (who later led the human genome sequencing project) at the University of Michigan. They had worked on discovering the gene responsible for the disease cystic fibrosis. Jim developed the gene therapy programme at the University of Pennsylvania from scratch. He hired many leading scientists in the areas of molecular biology, biochemistry, immunology, toxicology, pharmacology and related fields. The team worked hard to develop the OTC gene therapy product. I joined his team in 1996. I had gained my experience in studying immune responses to viruses such as HIV in humans.

The process of making a drug product using genes was a novel idea at that time. Gene therapy entails inserting a gene into the mutant cell. Technically it is extremely difficult to insert DNA into the nucleus of a cell and start expressing the protein. It was an amazing idea to utilize the unique properties of a virus to enter the cell. This property of the virus was harnessed by first removing the genes of the virus that were required for it to replicate. The viral gene was E1. The normal OTC gene was then stitched on to the E1-deleted adenovirus genome. This virus is now called a vector since it transports the OTC gene from outside the cell to the nucleus where it utilizes the cell's own machinery to enable the OTC gene to make the ornithine transcarbamylase enzyme. The hypothesis of the clinical trial was that expressing of the normal enzyme should correct the deficiency in a patient's liver.

After designing and developing the process to make the drug, extensive animal studies were performed. Genetically engineered mice that artificially had the OTC gene deleted were treated with the E1-deleted adenovirus vector. These mice were successfully treated for their OTC deficiency. The mice could process protein diets just like normal mice. The optimal dose required to treat the mice required extensive studies, which came under the field of pharmacology.

Pharmacology is the study of the distribution of a drug in the body (pharmacokinetics) and the effect of the drug on the body (pharmacodynamics). Many elegant experiments were performed to treat these OTC-deficient mice and the required dose was thus determined. The dose of the virus that cured the mice ranged from one to two million virus particles that expressed the normal OTC gene.

The next step in the development of a gene therapy drug to treat OTC gene deficiency was to study the side effects. This study is called toxicology. Normal rats and monkeys were given increasing doses of the drug to evaluate the maximum tolerated dose. The animals were monitored extensively for all their health parameters, including blood pressure, blood counts, and functions of the heart, liver and all tissues. Some of the animals were sacrificed so autopsies could be performed, and samples were taken from every organ to study the pathology that the drug may have caused. The findings showed that the drug had major side effects at higher doses and in fact may have resulted in the death of one monkey at this highest dose. The dose below this one was thus defined as the maximum tolerated dose. Under no circumstances should a human patient be subjected to a dose close to the maximum tolerated dose.

With the product characterized, (i.e. detailed physical and chemical analysis of the gene therapy product), pharmacology understood and the toxicity defined, the team submitted the application to initiate the clinical trial, called the investigational new product, to the FDA. Only after approval by the FDA can a clinical trial be initiated.

The first patient with OTC deficiency was dosed with the E1-deleted adenovirus vector expressing the normal OTC gene by injecting 2×10^9 virus particles that expressed the normal OTC gene into the vein that enters the liver directly.[*] This surgical procedure requires a catheter to guide the injection into the correct vein. Steve Raper, a surgeon who

---

[*] Raper, S.E., Chirmule, N., Lee, F.S., Wivel, N.A., Bagg, A., Gao, G.P., Wilson, J.M. and Batshaw, M.L. 'Fatal Systemic Inflammatory Response Syndrome in an Ornithine Transcarbamylase Deficient Patient Following Adenoviral Gene Transfer'. *Molecular Genetics and Metabolism* 80 (2003): 148–5.

had done hundreds of such procedures, administered the dose. The procedure went off without a glitch. Subsequently in the following months, seventeen patients with a confirmed OTC gene defect were given the drug with increasing doses. Jesse was patient number eighteen.

Jesse was admitted to the hospital and his blood tests performed before initiating the therapy. The vials that contained the vector were prepared in the manufacturing facility within the Hospital of the University of Pennsylvania. The manufacturing process followed the FDA guidelines described as good manufacturing practices (GMP). The quality department ensured that the vector preparation had passed all the tests required to ensure that the drug was indeed the E1-deleted adenovirus vector expressing OTC (identity), that it had no undefined impurities, and that it met all the predefined specifications for releasing the drug to be administered to the patient.

On 13 September 1999, the eighteenth patient, Jesse, was dosed. Steve Raper administered the drug to Jesse, after which there was a wait to see if it worked to express the normal OTC gene in Jesse's liver. About eighteen hours later, Jesse's speech became disturbed and his mental status seemed unstable. He had jaundice and all his organs—liver, heart and lungs—started to fail. There was inflammation in all his organs. The symptoms were similar to sepsis after an acute viral or bacterial infection. Medically, these symptoms are called disseminated intravascular coagulopathy, and multi-organ failure, which led to Jesse's death ninety-eight hours after the gene therapy was administered. Post-mortem evaluation confirmed that the virus vector had disseminated in most tissues. Blood samples taken at the time of death showed that there were abnormally high levels of proteins that had caused inflammation. These proteins included interleukin 6 and tumour necrosis factor alpha. Putting the clinical symptoms together with the laboratory findings suggested that Jesse may have died due to an over-activation of the immune response triggered by the adenovirus vector treatment.

The conclusions of the investigators led to findings that revealed several missteps during the process of drug development. Extensive investigation would have been required to study the relationship between dosage and inflammation. The toxicity studies could have been done in diseased animals rather than in normal animals, as required by the regulatory agencies. For example, one of the explanations of the dissemination of the virus vector (i.e. distribution of the virus after the injection) in Jesse's body is that it may have happened since his liver was already quite abnormal (fibrotic) due to several years of the disease. Biased decision-making and criminal and civil allegations against the management team of the trial resulted in a ban on Jim Wilson and the Institute for Human Gene Therapy from conducting future trials. It was a disastrous end to a trial that had started with the goal of treating a deadly disease and changing the course of medicine. But that was not to be at that time.

Many questions emerged. i) Why did Jesse die? ii) Was the scientific mechanism of the adverse reaction understood? iii) Could his death have been anticipated? iv) Did he die in vain? v) What was being done to ensure that deaths like Jesse's would not happen again? vi) Were there consequences to Jesse's death? vii) What is the accountability of the scientists and regulatory agencies in overseeing clinical trials like this?

While some of these questions have been answered, most people are not satisfied with the answers. But life must go on, and lessons must be learnt.

After the colossal failure of the OTC gene therapy trial, the FDA put a moratorium on all gene therapy trials. There was a major effort in the gene therapy community to come together and understand the science, ethics and safety of gene therapy trials. Until that time, most gene therapy trials had been done in academic hospital-based laboratories, where there may have been limited capabilities to develop high quality drugs and a lack of the infrastructure to manage the complex multi-departmental activities required for the treatment of patients. The latter is the forte of the biotechnology industry, which has efficient quality management systems to meet the standards of regulatory agencies, and regularly conducts clinical trials according to the guidelines and rules and regulations of the regulatory agencies.

The gene for OTC was delivered by inserting it into a virus, the adenovirus. This virus was used because of its ability to infect cells and chaperone the inserted gene into the cell. However, since the immune system 'sees' the virus as a foreign substance, it reacts violently. This inflammatory response was one of the reasons Jesse died.

With the lesson that adenovirus causes major immune side effects, there was an avalanche of research to discover and invent new ways to transfer genes into cells. Another virus, developed from a deep understanding of the biology of HIV (which is classified into a family of viruses called retroviral vectors), was engineered to make a transport system for genes. This virus vector carried the gene for another gene mutation, interleukin 2 receptor gamma chain (IL2Rγ). The absence or mutation of this gene in the bone marrow of children causes the immunological disease SCID, as we saw in the previous chapter.

Another group of scientists was quietly working away on a viral vector called adeno-associated virus, or AAV. It is a virus that does not cause any known disease. Its infectivity in humans is not high. Like all viruses, it requires the cellular machinery of the cells to replicate, express its proteins and grow. The viral DNA is a single strand and has to utilize the cell's nuclear engines to make a second strand. Arun Shrivastava, (Professor of Genetics, and Chief of Division of Cellular and Molecular Therapy at the University of Florida), Jude Samulski (Professor of Pharmacology at the University of Florida) and James Wilson (Professor of Medicine at the University of Pennsylvania) had been working on developing AAV as a vector for gene therapy. The advantages over the adenovirus were that it did not cause any known disease, it did not induce inflammatory immune responses, and it could infect non-dividing cells such as those of the muscle, brain and liver. The disadvantages were that it had a very small genome and therefore only a very small-sized gene could be inserted into the virus. The list of genes that could be inserted was therefore limited.

Jean Bennet, an ophthalmologist physician-scientist at the University of Pennsylvania, chose to insert a gene, the mutation of which causes progressive blindness.

Jean Bennet had closely watched the Jesse Gelsinger clinical trials. Jean is a very kind individual, unassuming and fiercely focused. She is an amazing mentor and has trained an extraordinary number of PhD and post-doctoral students, most of whom are now in major institutions across the world.

She and her husband are both ophthalmologists. While she has focused on conducting research, developing animal models and treating mice, dogs and monkeys, her husband has practised eye surgery. Jean was very interested in using gene therapy to treat a rare disease of the eye called retinitis pigmentosa. The disease is caused by a mutation in a gene called the retinitis pigmentosa esterase 65 (RPE65). She developed a method to insert the gene into AAV. She first tested the product to treat the same disease in dogs. The dog that was treated regained his vision. The trial was such a success that Congress wanted to see the dog for themselves. He was taken to Washington, D.C. to do a 'show-and-tell' session in the Capitol. With this proof-of-concept, it was time to test the product in humans.

All the lessons learnt from the previous clinical experiences with Jesse Gelsinger were studied and a detailed risk assessment and mitigation plan developed. All 'what if' scenarios were discussed, and the team was prepared to take on the challenge of treating human patients.

Unlike her predecessors, Jean's lab developed methods to insert the gene for RPE65 into AAV vectors made by a biotechnology company that was experienced in making medicines for patients. The gene therapy product that was made by Spark Biotechnology received approval for treatment of patients with retinitis pigmentosa using AAV-RPE65 gene therapy in 2018. It was shown to cure this form of blindness in humans. A huge success for the field, established on the lessons of past failures.

This success led to other trials.* Smooth muscular atrophy (SMA) is a form of muscular dystrophy. The defective gene in this disease is the dystrophin gene. The mutation results in a progressive loss of muscle function and mobility, which ultimately leads to heart and lung muscle function loss as well as challenges in swallowing. The incidence of the disease is one in 1,00,000. The mutation in this disease is on the survival motor neuron 1 (SMN1) gene,

---

* Daley, J. 'Gene Therapy Arrives: After False Starts, Drugs That Manipulate the Code of Life are Finally Changing Lives'. *Scientific American* (2020).

which encodes a protein that motor neurons need to survive. The mutation prevents this gene from producing that protein. The gene-targeting therapy, which was designed to express the normal SMN1 gene using the viral vector AAV, was developed by a small biotech company called AveXis. The company worked for decades on developing this drug and doing the proof-of-concept clinical studies. With the impressive results from their preclinical pharmacology studies, Novartis purchased AveXis for $8.7 billion in August 2018. They then conducted the clinical trials for FDA approval. The drug, called Zolgensma (onasemnogene abeparvovec-xioi), was approved for treatment of patients with SMA on 24 May 2019. In the trials, almost all the patients who received the one-time intravenous infusion of the high dose had rapid gains in motor functions, achieving major milestones associated with childhood development, including swallowing, rolling over and sitting independently, and a few could crawl or walk. This was an amazing accomplishment for the disease that had no treatment. While this treatment is not a complete cure for the disease, it is a huge step in the direction of providing hope for the future of treatment of genetic diseases. The cost of the drug is more than $2 million. The process of making this affordable requires the next generation of innovators.

The factors that contributed to the inflection point in the story of gene therapy are based on several research studies, each one contributing to one piece of the puzzle.

The scientific factors are: i) the discovery of DNA as the building blocks of all proteins (James Watson, Francis Crick and Rosalind Franklin); ii) the discovery of how proteins are made through ribosomes (Venki Ramakrishnan, Ada Yonath); iii) the discovery that mutations in a particular gene cause disease (Francis Collins and many others); iv) the recombinant DNA technology that enabled the insertion of a portion of DNA into the DNA of an organism (Genentech founders); v) the development of DNA technology to develop genetically modified animals (known as transgenic mice) that mimic the human disease so that the drug (the virus expressing the normal gene) can be tested for its efficacy; vi) the sequencing of the human genome (teams led by Francis Collins and Craig Venter); and vii) the ability to edit the genome to replace the mutated gene (Jennifer Doudna and Emmanuelle Charpentier).

Each one of these factors is a revolutionary finding in its own right, validated by the scientific community by awards, including the Nobel Prize. It is on the basis of discoveries and inventions like these that gene therapy will flourish. The lessons learnt in the operational aspects of clinical trials, i) the talent required to conduct such clinical studies, and ii) a culture of organizations* have many other factors that contribute to the inflection point that advances the field.

---

* Yohn, D.L. 'Company Culture is Everyone's Responsibility'. *Harvard Business Review*, 8 February 2021.

Successes/Failures

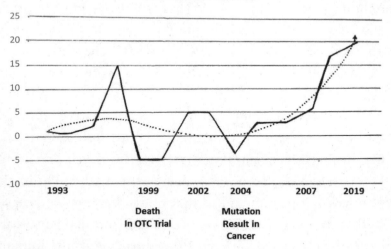

The specific events that take place are plotted as success or failures. The '0' line is the average.

Year	Event
1993	Adenoviral vectors are an efficient means to transfer genes
1998	Gene therapy is on an all-time high; several trials are under way
1999	Jesse Gelsinger dies
2002	Retroviral and lentiviral vectors, as well as adeno-associated (AAV) viral vectors are developed
2004	Insertional mutations result in causing cancer in boys treated with retroviral gene therapy
2007	The beginning of the refinement of AAV vectors
2019	AAV vectors are used to successfully treat patients with the eye disease retinitis pigmentosa and muscular atrophy disease

7

Biocon and My Own Story of Biotechnology

The art of combining technical and soft skills.

I had the unique opportunity to lead R&D at Biocon from 2015 to 2019.

I landed in Bangalore from Los Angeles on 5 May 2015, after having spent twenty-eight years in the US. Prior to moving to India, I was with Amgen, where I was Executive Director of Clinical Immunology. My extensive experience in studying the immunogenicity of vaccines and biologics and specifically interactions with regulatory agencies in the immunogenicity of biologics were my inflection points. Prior to my time with Amgen, I led the clinical immunology department at Merck Vaccines, and my experience in the clinical operations of large clinical trials, such as those for the rotavirus, HPV and zoster vaccines, was attractive to Amgen, which led them to recruit me. Before Merck, I had spent fifteen years in academia. I was at the University of Pennsylvania, where I did basic and applied research in the immunology of gene therapy, and at North Shore University Hospital, Cornell University Medical College, where I researched the pathogenesis of AIDS.

After almost three decades in the US and working for companies which focused on developing drugs for the US and developed countries, I was keen on working for a company that was developing drugs for developing and under-developed countries. I decided to make a major decision and work in India.

I joined Biocon as a result of a conversation with Kiran Mazumdar-Shaw. It was a chance meeting. My sister, Anjali, through her network, had connected me to Anita Fernandez, who was an administrative assistant to the Head of R&D at Biocon. She introduced me to the Abhijit Barve, and he invited me to give a talk on regulatory challenges in the development of biologics. After the talk, Kiran and I sat in the fine dining cafeteria at the Biocon campus in February 2015 and discussed my goals and her mission to make healthcare affordable. There was an immediate synergy. I then met a series of folks including Arun Chandavarkar (CEO), a serious and focused individual who had been the backbone of the operational aspects of the company for twenty-five years. Amit Saha (the head of HR), a warm person with high emotional intelligence, told me that 'We can learn a lot from you, from your years of experience in large pharma companies in the US'. In the coming years he would be a partner in studying, understanding and managing the culture of the organization. In the management team, I met Abhijit Barve, the head of R&D again and had a detailed conversation on the importance of immune responses in drug development. I had worked on immune responses to vaccines and biologics for three decades. A fun-loving and knowledgeable doctor, he had worked in various companies on developing generic drugs. He understood clinical operations well, which was the big gap for Biocon before he had arrived. He had done good work in developing a strong team to oversee clinical trials and clinical operations. I also met two amazing individuals in R&D, Dr Ramakrishnan Melarkode (Ramki) and Dr Nilanjan Sengupta. Both were responsible for developing the pharmacology aspects of the drug development process. I was impressed by their knowledge and understanding of this unique field. I considered myself an expert in this domain, having worked in this area across institutions for twenty-eight years. I knew they had done cutting-edge work in this field. These meetings sealed the deal for me to move to India after three decades in the US.

The other factors that led to my decision to relocate were: i) the association with family; ii) the access to amazing food; iii) the ability to further my musical aspirations (I had started learning dhrupad from my friend and guru, Tara Kini, and classical flute from Aditya Sutar); iv) the ability to travel within India; v) the chance to reconnect with long-lost friends; vi) the opportunity to contribute to social causes in India; and vii) the prospect of getting back to teaching. So on 5 May 2015, I boarded the British Airways flight from Los Angeles to Bangalore. My ex-wife Preeti, a rock-solid supporter of everything I have done in my career, dropped me off at the airport, patted my back, and said 'All the best'.

I joined Biocon on 5 May 2015. I did my orientation and had my introductory meeting. One of the first things I learnt was that Biocon had a major collaboration with Mylan. I had not heard of this company. Yes, I had not heard of one of the world's largest generics companies. That's how much I was in a cocoon in my career. But I learnt quickly that the collaboration between Biocon and Mylan was an important one for both companies as they brought their respective expertise to the table. The R&D scientists in Biocon have learnt the processes of making biologics, by expressing them in cells, and Mylan was a marketing giant, which had processes to market the drugs in many countries throughout the world, including the US and Europe.

In the collaboration I met and have made wonderful friends in both companies. Amazing people, amazing experiences, all working together for a common goal, of getting US FDA approval of the then biosimilar for trastuzumab, the antibody drug that binds to breast cancer cells and kills them. The original drug had been developed by Genentech/Roche, and its patent was running out. The biosimilar trastuzumab had to be similar to the original drug in its efficacy and safety. The guidelines and regulations for developing biosimilars were still being defined by the US-FDA. It took Biocon approximately eight years to develop this drug. The process of making this drug had been initiated before the Mylan collaboration. The long process involves designing the drug, manufacturing it, performing the pharmacology (i.e. how the drug works in the body to kill the tumour cells [pharmacodynamics], and how the body clears the drug [pharmacokinetics]), toxicology and clinical trials (figure below).

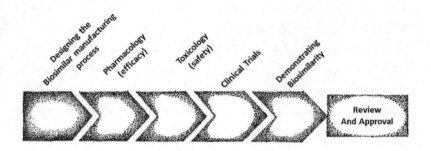

All the steps were completed. The million page biological licensing application (BLA) was submitted to the FDA for review.

It was noon on 1 December 2017 in Pittsburg. Barbara Militzer, who was the manager at Mylan, and led the regulatory interactions with the FDA, received an email from the FDA that the application for approval of the drug Ogivri for the treatment of breast cancer patients had been approved. Ecstasy. Nay, hysteria. She immediately sent an email to the management team of Biocon and Mylan, sharing this amazing news. Barbara was responsible for the communication between the Mylan-Biocon team working on Ogivri and the FDA.

She is a bubbly person with a lot of positive energy and was a major force behind the collaboration between the two companies. I was on that email, as the head of R&D at Biocon. I happened to be in Philadelphia that day with my daughter Anisha, and felt a huge sense of relief. The approval marked the culmination of a three-year journey at Biocon, and was the reward for all the ups and downs and lessons I had learnt during the past thirty years of my career. A US-FDA approval.

Obtaining the first approval of a bio-therapeutic drug (i.e., a class of drugs made in a biological system, and not by chemical reactions) by the US-FDA was a major milestone not just for Biocon, but for the biotechnology sector in India. It took more than two decades of extensive learning both in technology as well as in quality processes.

The story of biologics at Biocon started in 1999. The FDA defines biologics or biologic drugs as products made from living organisms or containing components of living organisms. The technical and regulatory pathway for developing biologics that were biosimilars* was not clear to the FDA itself. They were learning, experimenting and receiving advice from legislators, lobbyists, industries (the innovators and generics), professional associations, physicians and patients. The regulators were still in the process of understanding the requirements of establishing

---

* Biosimilars are biologics that are 'similar' to an approved biologic the patent for which has expired.

similarities between the reference product and the biosimilar. Despite this lack of clarity, what was crystal clear was that the investment for developing a biosimilar was going to be in the range of $100 million (approximately Rs 1000 crore). A huge investment. It was similar to the investment required to send the Chandrayaan rocket to space. It was a big risk to take. If there was a company in India to take on this challenge, it was Biocon. The courageous decision was made by management and the boards of the publicly traded companies, Mylan and Biocon. The collaborative team would develop the process to make biologic drugs since they have a huge impact on human health.

How does a company take such a big risk? What are the factors that it considers when undertaking such a formidable investment and such a Herculean task?

To answer these questions, it is critical to understand Biocon's journey.

Biocon has had innumerable inflection points in its growth trajectory since its inception in 1978. It is led by the legendary businesswoman, scientist and philanthropist Kiran Mazumdar-Shaw. She has an aura about her. She creates inflection points. Her influence on industries is much like the magic that Rajinikanth creates in his films; only hers is in real life. Her mere presence is sufficient to increase the value of a company and the value of the individual. My serendipitous meeting with her was my inflection point for my career and life.

Kiran started the journey of Biocon in 1978, when at the age of twenty-five she started making enzymes 'in the garage'. For a beautifully written story of Kiran and Biocon, I recommend *Mythbreaker: Kiran Mazumdar-Shaw and the Story of Indian Biotech*, by Seema Singh. I narrate below the abridged version, seen from my viewpoint.

In 1978, Kiran learnt beer-brewing in Australia. Due to societal disregard for hiring female brewmasters, she partnered with an Irish businessman to establish Biocon to make industrial enzymes.

Biocon began manufacturing and exporting papain, a plant enzyme, and isinglass, a marine hydrocolloid, which are key products for the beer brewing industry, in a small factory in Bangalore. The company very quickly established a leadership position in developing enzymes using fermentation technologies and was supported by various investors including Unilever. In 1999, Biocon sold the enzyme business to Novozymes and switched its focus to developing biological pharmaceutical drugs. This decision was a major inflection point for the company. It worked on developing processes to manufacture small molecule generics (drugs whose patents have expired) using fermentation technologies rather than medicinal chemistry processes; a decision that in retrospect was another inflection point for the company.

Another important decision was to develop affordable medicines. Pursuing this mission entailed big investments, building large facilities and leveraging economies of scale for competitive pricing. This, Biocon did successfully.

Today, thanks to the huge undertaking by several investors, and the efforts of mentoring board members and thousands of loyal employees and well-wishers, Biocon is one of the largest manufacturers of statins and limus drugs in the world. Statins—such as lovastatin, simvastatin, atorvastatin, pravastatin and rosuvastatin—are a class of drugs that help reduce cholesterol and thus save the lives of millions of people by preventing heart attacks and strokes. Limus drugs such as tacrolimus and everolimus are used in controlled suppression of the immune system in patients undergoing organ and bone marrow transplants. (Incidentally, my friend Murali takes tacrolimus to ensure the kidney transplant he received from his brother is not rejected.)

These drugs have impacted billions of lives, which is why this statement of the company's mission rings loud: 'To make drugs and medicines affordable to all, with an innovation model seeking to "reduce disparities in access to safe, high-quality medicines, as well as address the gaps in scientific research to find solutions to impact a billion lives".'*

Many pharmaceutical companies in India developed innovative chemical engineering processes for active

---

* https://www.mckinsey.com/featured-insights/asia-pacific/why-a-cut-and-paste-approach-to-digital-transformation-wont-cut-it-an-interview-with-the-founder-of-biocon#

pharmaceutical ingredients (APIs) and formulations, which has resulted in these companies becoming among the largest providers of generic drugs across the world under the abbreviated new drug application (ANDA) regulatory process. Cipla, Sun Pharma, Aurobindo, Dr. Reddy's and Intas are just some of these companies. For the decade 2000–10, the generic drug development industry in India has streamlined the processes of scale up and regulatory inspections, resulting in approvals. Estimates indicate that approximately 40 per cent of all the small pharmaceutical drugs in the US are made in part by an Indian company. Biocon played its part in contributing to this success.

Were there challenges in the development and approval of drugs by the international regulatory agencies? Of course. This journey was not easy. Katherine Eban has written about the wrongdoings of some companies in India in her book *Bottle of Lies: The Inside Story of the Generic Drug Boom*. It is a scathing account, but this story does not represent most Indian pharmaceutical companies, especially Biocon. The emphasis on quality systems and the focus on developing a culture of quality in the organization are important. This culture is seen in most companies in India today. Are we perfect? Absolutely not. Are we improving every day? Absolutely. The future will see a transformation in the quality and affordability of medicine.

2004 was a landmark year for Biocon, financially. The company needed to raise Rs 300 crore to fund its ambitious capital expansion plans. Public funding was the option. The initial public offering (IPO) in March 2004 was oversubscribed thirty-two times. Biocon closed day one of listing with a market value of $1.11 billion to become only the second Indian company to cross the $1 billion mark on the day of listing. Money was now available to develop drugs. *What bold decisions would Biocon make next?*

Insulin, a drug, our natural hormone (a biologic), was first approved almost a century ago, in 1900. That insulin was purified from the pancreas of dogs. It took another eighty years for the science of recombinant DNA technology (described in Chapter 1 for factor VIII), to be invented. In early 1980s, Genentech first, then Novo Nordisk, Sanofi and Eli Lilly pioneered the development of insulin as a drug, thanks to which diabetes was no longer a disease with a death sentence but rather a lifestyle chronic disease. In India, however, it was only in early 2000, that Biocon decided to pursue the development and manufacturing of insulin. After a few years of developing the process and testing in clinical trials, insulin was approved by the Indian regulatory body, CDSCO, in 2004. This approval was a landmark event for India in the history of insulin as a drug. Approval of Biocon Insulin in India had a dramatic effect in terms of lowering the pricing due to competition.

How did Biocon make insulin that had such a large effect of affordability, and why did it take so many years? Let's look at the situation in Biocon in the late 1990s.

The leadership at Biocon made a bold decision to express the insulin gene in yeast, called *Pichia pastoris*. *Why was this decision such a remarkable one?* The seven reasons below outline the story of insulin development in Biocon.

First was the factor of internal expertise. To develop a biologics drug, one of the major tenets in Biocon is to utilize the capabilities and expertise within the company. Since the team at Biocon had deep experience in developing processes to make products using fermentation of bacterial and biological organisms, growing *Pichia pastoris* fell in the sweet spot of Biocon's bioengineering expertise. The bioengineering team was led by Arun Chandavarkar. Arun had a PhD from MIT in bioengineering and expertise in manufacturing processes. Biocon also has a fantastic, loyal and long-tenured team, including Shreehas Tambe (UDCT, Mumbai; twenty years with Biocon), Shrikumar Suryanarayanan (IIT-Madras; twenty-five years), Harish Iyer (IIT-Madras; ten years), Anuj Goel (NCL, Pune; twenty years), Ramakrishnan Melarkode (IIS, Bangalore; twenty years), Partha Hazra (University of California, San Diego; twenty years), Karthik Ramani (State University of New York, Rochester; twenty years), Anand Khedkar (ICT Mumbai, ~ten years), Ankur Bhatnagar (IIT-Delhi; twenty years), Jyoti Iyer (Indian Institute of Chemical Technology [ICT], previously University Department of Chemical Technology [UDCT] Mumbai; twenty years) and Laxmi Adhikary (Banaras Hindu University; twelve years), among many others.

The *second* contributing factor was the physical facility. Kiran and her team had shown great foresight in purchasing a vast tract of land for the Biocon campus, which spreads over an expanse of about 100 acres. In addition, Biocon invested $161 million in 2011 to build a large manufacturing facility in Iskandar, Johor, Malaysia. Biocon could therefore set up the manufacturing sites required to produce large amounts of insulin, measured in tonnes of protein. The team was also able to establish the quality management systems to support GMP that are required for regulatory approval.

The *third* factor was market need. Diabetes is widespread in India as well as around the world. Control of diabetes with insulin is central to the management of the late stages of this deadly disease. There was a desperate need to make available affordable insulin for patients. The scientific and financial considerations of calculating and mathematical modelling of the financial considerations of expenses and income, and market need determines the value of the product. The net present value (NPV) was positive.

The *fourth* was cost of the competition. In 2004, the cost of insulin in India was a few thousand rupees. Very few people could afford it. Designing a manufacturing process using the *Pichia pastoris* expression system was key to bringing down the cost.

Fifth was the technical opportunity of a platform to make other products using *Pichia pastoris*. Novo Nordisk makes insulin using another strain of yeast, Saccharomyces, while Eli Lilly manufactures it by means of E. coli bacteria.

The decision to use *Pichia pastoris* was based on Biocon's expertise in understanding the genome and therefore having the ability to systematically manipulate the genes, the understanding of the biochemistry, and the availability of appropriate technology to develop a process to meet business requirements.

The *sixth* factor was related to environment—political, social and economic. With the opening of financial markets in India, the signing of the World Trade Organization treaty, and consumer confidence in modern medicines, it was an opportune time to launch insulin.

And *finally*, there was the pride of 'make in India' and a deep focus on quality. The small molecule industry in India had matured and the country was fast on its way to becoming the 'pharmacy of the world', providing APIs for a wide variety of drugs. Although the 'Make in India' brand was not launched till much later, the pride of innovation in India had taken seed. Biocon played and continues to play a major role on this front.

All the factors noted above favoured the decision to express the protein in the novel vector, *Pichia pastoris*. Insulin was approved under the brand name Insugen, and a couple of years later, a device used for injecting the insulin, Insupen, was introduced. Today, in addition to Biocon, several other companies in India manufacture insulin including Wockhardt and Torrent. The ultimate benefactor in this technology-driven enterprise is the patient. The price of insulin has dropped from several thousand rupees to a few hundred rupees per day for a diabetic patient who needs to take an injection every day. In 2019, Kiran announced at the UNAIDS Health Innovation Exchange in New York, 'Biocon will make its recombinant human insulin available at less than ten cents per day in low- and middle-income countries. These countries contribute to 80 per cent of the global diabetes burden. In comparison, the current US list price in retail is more than $5 a day or more.'

A different set of technologies is required to develop biologics, namely, expression of proteins by recombinant technologies and use of fermentation technologies. Given the success with insulin, Biocon decided to delve further into the manufacturing of biologics and biosimilars. There is a very interesting and fascinating back story to the introduction of biologics to Biocon.

In 1999, after a serendipitous interaction with scientist from Cuba, Kiran licensed a novel asset, itolizumab, to develop a drug for the treatment of psoriasis. Cuban scientists at the Centre of Molecular Immunology (CIM) had worked on this molecule, itolizumab, for several years. Since the US had imposed sanctions on Cuba, American companies could not work with their immediate neighbours, and scientists in Cuba could not develop the drug for most countries in the world. Hence it was opportune for Kiran to strike a deal with the Cuban institute. Scientists such as Eduardo Montero in Cuba had developed technologies to manufacture recombinant proteins. Their kindness towards the folks at Biocon, and 'wanting to give and sharing the knowledge of development of biologics' attitude were exemplary. They were instrumental in training the Biocon team on the fundamentals of developing biologic drugs, from molecular cloning of genes into stable cell lines, growing these cells in bioreactors (termed upstream process) and purifying the product by removing impurities of the cell debris material (termed downstream process) to formulation. In 2006, the process enabled the development and successful launch of a novel monoclonal antibody by Biocon, targeting the epidermal growth factor receptor (EGFR) for the treatment of colorectal cancer and cancer of the head and neck, Biomab-EGFR, was approved by the Indian regulator, CDSCO. (Vectibix and Erbitux, biologics targeting the EGFR by Amgen and Eli Lilly, respectively, obtained approvals in 2006 and 2009.) And then, in 2013, another novel monoclonal antibody targeting the CD6 molecules on T cells, Alzumab, developed for treating plaque psoriasis, was approved in India. Biocon was on a roll in developing novel biologics, at par with biotechnology majors such as Amgen, Genentech and Eli Lilly.

Then why did Biocon not pursue the development of novel biologics at the pace of the Amgens of the world?

To answer this question, let us use the analogy of children going to school. A child first goes to elementary school, then middle school and on to high school, after which comes college. This is followed by one's first job, and so on. With the Cubans arriving in Bangalore to work on biologics and train the scientists in India, Biocon had entered elementary school with respect to learning the biologics process. The process of obtaining approvals for Alzumab® and Biomab® in India provided learning to the scientists at Biocon, with hand-holding from the Cubans, the equivalent of middle school. The next stage, high school and college, would require exponential learning. Amgen had been developing biologics since 1998; it was therefore already in college. (Reminder: Biocon had developed small molecules from 1999 to 2009.) Biocon needed to go to high school before going to college. High school for Biocon was the development of biosimilars. For this effort, it needed another partner. A marriage with Mylan.

To demonstrate the growth of understanding for the scientists in Biocon over time, I continue to use the analogy of graduating from school to college, as advances are made in approvals of more complex class of drugs. Small molecule generics—Biologics (monoclonal antibodies) to Biosimilars. Biocon had at least three inflection points leading to the success of the first approval for biosimilars.

The first inflection point was approvals for small molecules, Biocon could leverage these technologies of fermentation processes, since most of the generic small molecule products, such as the limus class of small-molecule drugs for immunosuppressants and statins, were developed using similar fermentation and purification processes. Biocon's experience with fermentation provided a natural transition to developing biologics. Biosimilars were developed by reverse engineering the reference product, made by the originator company.

The second inflection point was the Cuban connection. The scientist from Cuba spent several years in the Biocon research laboratories in Bangalore training the team on processes to manufacture and characterize Biologics. This experience was established by the regulatory approvals of monoclonal antibody drugs, such as BioMab (for the treatment of colon cancer) and Alzumab (for the treatment of psoriasis).

The third inflection point was provided the collaboration with the Mylan team, who brought a wealth of diverse experiences from operational processes, regulatory strategy, and also by my own experience in working with the FDA through consortiums. These experiences proved to be very useful in understanding the complex processes of the work to be done and its alignment with the regulatory path. We connected with the FDA folks I had known for many years to advise us on how to navigate the regulatory path. Another unexpected thing happened. Dozens of my dear friends, a majority of whom had done their education in India, and now had high ranking positions in various institutions in the US, were eager to give advice to my colleagues in Biocon. This advice offered crucial learnings to solve extremely difficult challenges, that would otherwise have taken several months and years to solve. This support gave us the confidence that we were not flying blind.

Let's get back to the process of making biosimilar drugs. It's not easy; in fact one could make a case, sometimes it is more difficult than a novel drug. To understand the process of making a biosimilar drug, let us use the analogy of football. The goal of the game is to kick the ball into the goal precisely and accurately. The size of the goal is fixed. In the case of a reference product, each manufacturing lot has some amount of variability. It is never exactly the same. Several lots are obtained from the market and tested for their ability to perform the desired function. In the case of trastuzumab, it was its ability to kill breast cancer tumour cells. Trastuzumab biosimilar was chosen to be developed, since the patent for exclusivity was expiring. The competition is stiff, since many big companies in the world, including Amgen, Pfizer, Merck, with extensive resources, were also developing this biosimilar drug. The variability in the potency of each lot defines the size of the goal post. In other words, the range of acceptable variability, such that despite the variation, each lot is effective in killing the tumour cells. With the size of the goal post set, Biocon developed a process to manufacture biosimilar trastuzumab so that each lot manufactured would kill the breast cancer cells in a 'similar' range as the reference product. In the analogy, each shot at the goal should cross the goal post. As long as the ball goes through the goal post 95 per cent of the time, the regulators accept biosimilarity.

Now, let's translate the analogy to the science of biosimilars.

Establishing biosimilarity (i.e., demonstrating that the biosimilar project is equivalent to the reference drug in safety and efficacy) requires a systematic approach by first understanding each 'component of the drug'; in scientific lingo, 'the critical quality attributes of the molecules'. When one analyses the structure of the protein drug, it has several features such as: physico-chemical including protein-sequence, sugars associated with the protein, the way it folds in solution, etc. There are more than forty different analytical methods to measure these features of the drug. Using these analytical methods, several batches of the biosimilar product need to be compared with several batches of the reference product. The two products should be 'similar'. Similarity is established using sophisticated statistical methods. The emphasis on demonstrating analytical similarity is the first step in the biosimilarity process.

Following a demonstration of analytical similarity, equivalence with the biological function of the reference product required pharmacokinetic (the effect of the body on the drug) and pharmacodynamic (effect of the drug on the body) clinical studies, which are powered for equivalence, and the ranges using variability of the end point measurements previously used by the reference product. The criteria for establishing equivalence were established on the principles of the International Council for Harmonization of Technical Requirements for Pharmaceuticals for Human Use (ICH) Q5E. This process is defined by regulatory agencies across the world, and the similarity of the biosimilar drug and reference product needs to be demonstrated unequivocally. The detailed analysis of eight years of work in developing the process and demonstrating biosimilarity is summarized by a report by the US FDA.[*]

After establishing biosimilarity by analytical testing and clinical trials, the manufacturing process to produce the biosimilar needs to be established, and audited for quality by the regulatory agencies. Establishing a robust quality controlled process for manufacturing requires a large number of people to work in a highly organized manner to ensure each lot of the product meets the quality standard established during process development. The management of such a highly regulated, constantly audited manufacturing process requires commitment, dedication, focus, and a high level of integrity.

Katherine Eban's book *Bottle of Lies* provides a scathing account of the generics industry. Lack of attention to detail affects the quality of processes, which can result in defective products. In medicine, every pill, every injection and every device counts. It affects lives. It takes a concerted

---

[*] FDA Briefing Document, Oncologic Drugs Advisory Committee Meeting, 13 July 2017, BLA 761074 MYL-1401O, 'A Proposed Biosimilar to Herceptin (trastuzumab)', https://www.fda.gov/media/106566/download. Accessed on 12 May 2021.

effort across various functions in an organization to come together with the common purpose of ensuring quality.

After I joined Biocon in 2015 as head of R&D, I quickly realized that it was not the science nor the talented scientists, but robust processes that would be central to achieving approval by the US FDA. Many, if not most companies in India have processes that are people-dependent; in fact society at large is people-dependent. If you need to get any major task done, you need to know someone in a key position! Isn't it? Robust manufacturing requires a process-dependent culture, where automation, digitization and data analytics can play a big role in ensuring failures do not occur. Of course, people are required, but the process should not be dependent on them. Changing the culture of an organization from a people-oriented to process-oriented one is a difficult task.

To understand the culture of quality systems in operations, let us take the hypothetical example of a manufacturing facility where there is an extremely clean fill-finish operation of filling vials, capping and labelling. *What is the qualification of the person who is responsible for cleaning the facility?* This person is from a village, probably educated only till high school, and on the low end of the economic scale. The Tyvek gown that must be worn before entering the facility is likely more expensive than the clothes he wears. He must change into this gown every day and discard it when he leaves the facility. One day, as he comes out of the facility and throws his expensive gown into the trash, he realizes that he has left his favourite pen inside the facility. He does not want to 'waste' company money and so enters the facility without donning a new Tyvek gown, because it will 'just take one second to pick up the pen and quickly run out'. He does that. The camera in the room records this event. During the regulatory inspection, this event is noted. The site gets a warning letter. Or worse, the $200-million facility is shut down due to lack of procedures and training.

So, the question is, how can this situation be avoided? By extensive and continuous training. Most importantly, the training should ensure each employee understands why the procedures in place must be followed to the T. This type of training, which enhances a person's soft skills, is not as easy as it sounds. Highly experienced trainers are required to do this job. It is not just a checklist approach to training.

Imparting such training entails understanding the mindset of the individual being trained. Where does he live? How does he live? He lives with meagre resources. The environment he lives in requires him to struggle through crowded streets, unruly traffic and the ordered chaos of life in a typical Indian city. He enters the gates of the manufacturing facility and is suddenly in a completely different world. A world where everything is (supposed to be) in order. He must follow all the standard operating procedures. Every deviation must be recorded. The two worlds he inhabits are as different as night and day. The training processes should address the cultural differences of this dichotomy. Understanding the cultures of organizations and workplaces, as well as work-life balance, should be an integral part of training programmes.

Among the many aspects of establishing a quality controlled process in an organization, training of the staff is a critical component. Training staff includes developing a continuous training process, ensuring that the training is relevant, and that the trained personnel have understood the training. Regulatory agencies audit the training processes of an organization.

Biocon received approval for the biosimilar trastuzumab on 1 December 2017. It was a monumental day for the nearly forty-year-old company. The team had done everything that was required to get this approval: the science, the process, the trainings, and most importantly, the quality.

What lessons did we learn from the US FDA approval of biosimilar trastuzumab?

To deconvolute the learnings from the decade of work, from 2009–19, and apply it to the mission of the company of 'making affordable healthcare', we need to understand the details. Let us go back a decade, to 2009.

The lessons learnt in this process of developing biosimilars can be categorized under: i) the organizational structure; ii) the process of solving difficult problems; iii) operational efficiencies; and iv) regulatory strategies.

i)   The organizational structure:

As Head of R&D, there were several tasks, all of which were high priority for the company, that needed to be completed. (I was drinking water from a fire hose!) Hence, the first task was to develop a strong, and well-coordinated team to evaluate what worked and what did not. We needed to identify someone who could help in working both with the junior teams, and also with senior management. That someone turned out to be Monalisa Chatterji, Associate Director, a highly driven young leader, who was not afraid to tell the facts as they were. She was one of the folks who had spent time in the US (at Yale University) and hence was experienced in a different culture. It was not the purpose of the team to develop a culture 'like the US', but rather a culture that was required for Biocon to succeed. In order to understand the various activities that were required to prepare the team for the enormous task of submitting a high-quality data set for obtaining US FDA approval, we needed to prioritize the tasks. *Thus, what lessons from drug development were relevant for Biocon?* We needed to anticipate all the risks before they occurred; conduct an in-depth analysis of all the potential things that could go wrong; list their causes; define the effects; and take actions. This process is termed failure mode and effect analysis. We initiated the process of reviewing the long list of risks at offsites.

It became immediately clear that the scientific leadership team was doing much more than was required, and a centralized prioritization was required. Classically, biotechnology companies are organized by function. Each function is like a department in an academic institution. The leaders in these groups had grown organically through the ranks in the company. Was it necessary to change the leadership? I came from organizations that made changes to leadership every two to three years. Which was the better decision for Biocon?

ii) The process of solving difficult problems:

May 2015. Everyone was in high spirits. The Gantt charts made by project management for submission of the dossier was showing the third quarter of 2017. The process for manufacturing the trastuzumab biosimilar product at a commercial scale had been developed. More than thirty different extremely sophisticated analytical tests that were required to characterize the product, were in the process of being developed and then validated. Jyoti Iyer was leading a highly cross-functional team. There was a sense of urgency. We were trying to figure out the specific steps of developing Biocon's first biologics drug for approval by the US FDA. It was a daunting task. While the process from submission to approval was described in manuals and guidelines by the US FDA, and the necessary standards were defined by United States Pharmacopeia, doing it in real-time was another matter. So many steps had to be done in parallel. The product had to be manufactured at a scale that would precisely define the commercial process; clinical trials had to be conducted; the analytical testing of ten different lots of the product made at commercial scale had to be done to establish similarity with the reference product; the stability of the product had to be demonstrated in time-course studies, where the product was stored in different conditions, and tested to determine if it did not degrade. In these experiments the product was subjected to high temperatures and forced to degrade; and biological tests are done to demonstrate stability in these conditions, which can be experienced when the drug is shipped to different parts of world. It was indeed a complex, multi-step, highly cross-functional process.

Anything in this process could go wrong, and it always does. There has to be a process to anticipate the potential problem (risk assessment), and a process to solve the problem (and investigative corrective action process)

iii) Operational efficiencies:

In Biocon, it clearly was not a well-oiled machine at that time. It was the first time a biologic was being developed. Many activities were uncoordinated. Weekly meetings were conducted to oversee each team's activities to ensure nothing slipped through the cracks. These meetings allowed the teams to understand how each team was connected to the others. All wheels needed to work together, and anything one team did affected another. The team that performed the analytical testing of the product was required by all the other teams, such as process development teams, pharmacology teams, toxicology teams and clinical teams. This analytical team was common to most teams, since any process needs to measure the activities. Many of the incidents that were encountered were tackled through specific teams, and solved. If the incidents were of a larger magnitude, they would involve other teams, and the entire 'engine' of development of the drug would stall.

One of the incidents that arose had to do with the process of filling the product into vials. This process involves taking the bulk material and adding precise amounts in a vial in a manufacturing facility that fills millions of vials in a few hours. The amount of product that was being filled in a vial was exceeding that defined by the specifications by only a fraction of a millilitre. That extra amount was sufficient for the product to not be similar to the reference product. Anything different (less or more), outside an acceptable variance, and the biosimilar product may not have the same therapeutic value as the reference product. *How does one solve this problem?*

It requires a deep understanding of every step in the process of filling each vial on the assembly line. One must ascertain what factors contribute to the variability, and then develop a control process to ensure the accuracy of the fill. A risk assessment step is also required to anticipate what conditions would enable the filling to be accurate. Brilliant statistical modelling work and risk analysis by Karthik Ramani, who led the product formulation and stability groups, enabled the accuracy of this process. Karthik is an extremely knowledgeable scientist who trained at the University of New York at Albany in the US. One of his hobbies is playing the mridangam, and the skills he had developed while mastering this art no doubt helped solve this sticky issue.

Another difficult problem. Proteins are glycosylated: Glycosylation is the process of adding carbohydrates to proteins inside the cells. Carbohydrates are added to proteins inside the endoplasmic reticulum and Golgi organelles of the cells. Glycosylation is an extremely sophisticated process that enables proteins to become stable, fold correctly and perform their functions with a high degree of specificity and efficiency.

The Chinese Hamster Ovary (CHO) cells, in which the antibody drug is being made, induce glycosylation in a particular manner wherein the precise conditions that result in specific enzymes being activated orchestrate the final product. The enzymes and the culture conditions that resulted in the glycosylation of the trastuzumab made by Roche, which first made the molecule, would naturally be different from the one we were trying to make. How much difference in the glycosylation profile the protein made by Biocon would make the product function (i.e., ability to kill breast-cancer cells) differently enough to that of the reference product? Anushikha Thakur, a feisty young PhD scientist who was trained in high-end analytical techniques at the Indian Institute of Science, Bangalore, and Pradeep Kabadi, who had been with Biocon for more than ten years and was an expert in analytical techniques, were tasked with the analysis of the glycan patterns of the Biocon product and the reference product under the oversight of Ramki.

Mass spectrometry is an extremely sensitive technique to measure the range of different kinds of sugar molecules (isoforms) of these glycans. There are thirteen different forms of glycan proteins that can be distinctly separated, and their relative amounts calculated. The results showed that while the major isoforms were within a 20 per cent variable range, there were a few minor glycans that were slightly different. The nature of these differences and their potential impact on the function of the molecule were debated extensively in numerous internal meetings. After all, if the glycosylations in the biosimilar product and reference product were significantly different, the Biocon product would not be considered a biosimilar. A lot was at stake.

A crack team was formed to solve this incident. The team consisted of Anushikha and Pradeep's physico-chemical scientists; biological scientists led by Harish Pai; and bioanalytical scientists led by Nilanjan Sengupta. Both Harish and Nilanjan had been with Biocon for over ten years and had extensive experience in the biological aspects of the product, as well as the ability to address challenging scientific problems. The team performed extensive structure-function analyses of the various isoforms of the glycosylated product using purified proteins tested in cell culture and concluded that the differences observed in the glycosylation patterns between the Biocon-made product and the reference product were not functionally different. More than a year later, the FDA also reviewed these analyses during the audit process, agreed with the conclusions and approved the product as a biosimilar. This kind of analysis, problem-solving and teamwork is the 'day job' of a scientist in a pharmaceutical company.

iv) Regulatory strategies:

On 1 December 2016, the one-million-page document detailing the entire development story of biosimilar trastuzumab was submitted to the FDA by the Mylan regulatory team. It was the culmination of eight years of blood and sweat and a labour of love.

The events in the year 2017, related to interacting with the US FDA regulators, provided the most profound learning experiences for the entire team—R&D, quality control, regulatory activities, intellectual property, finance, business, marketing and management. It was the first application for a biologic from either Biocon or Mylan; it was also the first biosimilar trastuzumab package submitted to the FDA. (The Biocon–Mylan team had beaten the odds and submitted their package before the heavyweight competition, namely, Amgen–Allergen and Merck–Samsung.) The FDA appoints an advisory committee to review the first application of approval of drugs. This committee comprised experienced clinicians, data management experts, statisticians, nurses, regulatory and quality professionals. There were sixteen external reviewers and four FDA observers. The date for the review meeting had been set for 13 July 2017. The Biocon–Mylan team had six months to prepare. The process of preparing for such an advisory committee (Ad-Comm) review entails the most extensive work that an R&D organization will ever do to get approval for a drug. I was fortunate to have been through that process four times before. This time, I was leading the effort for Biocon. It was a huge responsibility.

More than fifty scientists from Biocon had critical information for their respective departments. Those who would be presenting the material to the committee were chosen based on their oration skills, experience and most importantly, ability to take the pressure of the moment. Arnd Annweiler, head of R&D at Mylan (my counterpart), who trained as a molecular biologist at the University of Heidelberg, Germany, was to do the introduction. Patrick Vallano, who headed the bioanalytical group, described the non-clinical work. Finally, Abhijit Barve, head of clinical development at Mylan, presented the safety and efficacy results of the clinical trials. Between January and July 2017, the Biocon team made eight trips to Washington, D.C. for face-to-face prep meetings. Jyoti Iyer, Ramki Melarkode, Rajshekhar Vanga (who headed the regulatory group) and I were in the core team. Fifty-three scientists at Biocon were part of this once-in-a-lifetime opportunity of preparing for an FDA advisory committee. Several hundred others watched the prep proceedings by video.

The team went through at least five thousand tough questions that were posed by the external consultants, cross-functional teams and regulatory experts. Each question had a detailed answer.

This was the college education for Biocon.

Finally, the day of the committee meeting dawned— 13 July 2017. It was to be held at the FDA offices in Silver Springs, Washington, D.C.

At 11 a.m., a shiny black Mercedes-Benz forty-seater bus arrived at the hotel where the Biocon–Mylan team was staying. The forty team members, each dressed in formals, boarded the bus. The bus arrived at the FDA office, and the team went through the security check, everyone displaying their passports, which were from various countries, including India, Italy, Germany, England, China, Philippines and the US. The team members took their respective positions in the conference room; the speakers sat near the podium; the twenty experts who had prepared the potential answers to questions sat in the 'pit'; and the remaining, including me, sat in the audience. It reminded me of a court of law. In fact, it was. The FDA approval depended upon the quality of the presentation, which represented all the work done through the course of the drug manufacturing process.

The proceedings began. Arnd started, followed by Patrick, and then Abhijit. Their presentations were crisp and clear, as they had practiced hundreds of times. Questions ensued. About 2000 slides had been prepared to help answer any questions that might arise. The review went on for two hours. When the questions were finally done, it was time for the vote. The chairperson (judge) asked the committee (jury) to vote for a recommendation of approval. The vote was a unanimous 'yes'. There was silence for almost a minute. I was jumping with joy in my mind, but remained quiet and calm on the outside.

The announcement of the approval was made matter-of-factly. The FDA Oncology Drug Advisory Committee unanimously recommended the approval of the Biocon–Mylan proposed biosimilar trastuzumab. Based on the data presented on the results of the manufacturing process, and the non-clinical and clinical studies, the members of the committee voted 16:0 in support of the treatment of patients with breast cancer with this drug.

In the coming weeks, the FDA conducted a detailed review of the million pages of the dossier and had more than 10,000 questions. Rajshekhar Vanga, Chetan Sharma, Rekha N. and the regulatory team along with their Mylan counterparts responded in detail to these questions. Sriram Akundi, Biocon's head of quality, and his Mylan counterparts fronted the audits and fielded the questions on quality management systems.

And on 1 December 2017, Barbara Militzer received the email informing the team of the FDA approval.

Of course, the lessons I had learnt in the thirty years of my career in drug development helped, but such a huge accomplishment cannot be achieved by one person. A huge thank you to the amazing team at Biocon and Mylan, without whom this would never have happened.

As a result of the approval, trastuzumab became affordable; the impact of this is huge. There is also a place for biosimilars to enhance competition and make drugs affordable.

Biocon had graduated from college.

Appendix

Kiran Mazumdar-Shaw has been a colleague, boss, friend and mentor to me. I first met Kiran in February 2015. Her charisma and ability to clearly articulate complex social and technical issues and translate them into practical aspects is her strength. She is focused on making healthcare affordable and accessible. She is persistent and has endless energy to work on diverse projects, such an overseeing a multibillion-dollar company, being on the boards of other major companies and internationally acclaimed academic institutions, mentoring young entrepreneurs, working with the government on health policies, and so much more. Each of these interactions has a purpose, to feed her passion. Yet, she is approachable and just a phone call away. Her ability to toggle high pressure work with her extraordinary social calendar is something I have tried to learn how to do.

Appendix

The following are some memorable quotes

'I think, in terms of corporate philosophy, I've always believed that you've got to treat people in a very, very egalitarian manner in the sense I like to treat people on a one-to-one basis. And I like people to take on a lot of responsibilities because I think with a sense of responsibility also comes a sense of purpose.'

'I really believe that entrepreneurship is about being able to face failure, manage failure and succeed after failing.'

'You have to build a culture of philanthropy. In a country like India, we need to be sensitive and caring about the poorer, more disadvantaged section of our country.'

'Today anything can be done—we have the techniques.'

'I hate the title of being called "the richest woman in India", but it's the recognition that this was the value that I had created as a woman entrepreneur, and that makes me very, very proud.'

'I do serve on various boards and I'm very honest and frank, obviously. I am a very forthright person and I do, sort of, share my candid views on anything.'

'My legacy is going to be in affordable healthcare. I am willing to invest in developing that model and the policies around it.'

'One of my objectives when I started Biocon was to make sure that I create a company for women scientists to pursue a vocation.'

'An entrepreneur's life is always a continuous journey.'
'I learnt that business was about being emotionally driven about investing, but being emotionally detached when it came to divesting and that's a very strong learning.'

The people

Anuj Goel, a quiet, intense man with a no-nonsense attitude, had been with Biocon for more than twenty years. He has a PhD in process development from Pune's National Chemical Laboratory. Anuj and I had a very interesting relationship. We rarely talked about anything outside of work. I respected his advice, especially his insights regarding people in the company, which helped me develop organizational strategies that required key folks in key positions.

Ramakrishnan Melarkode, or Ramki, was head of analytical sciences at Biocon. He was a very colourful person. Highly motivated and loyal, he had also been with Biocon for more than twenty years. He was highly respected for his encyclopaedic knowledge about the work being done in the field. He was also knowledgeable about a wide variety of subjects, from Tourette's syndrome, ribosomes and cytokines to history and art.

Both Ramki and Anuj were the backbones of the R&D organizational structure.

Jyoti Iyer is an ambitious leader with great self-confidence and knowledge. She has the great ability to help people in their time of need. Outside of work, she is deeply involved with an organization that helps underprivileged children. With her colleagues she has rented a house on the outskirts of Bangalore and raised funds to support the schooling and cultural activities of twenty-five children.

At work, Jyoti was responsible for the development of the manufacturing process of drugs that involved purification and removal of impurities. Utilizing her knowledge of separation techniques, she and her group optimized the process to purify the trastuzumab biosimilar product such that there were minimal impurities. The smallest amount of impurity could potentially lead to major side effects ranging from skin reactions to inflammation and even death (due to anaphylactic shock). I had had experience with most of these disasters during the course of my career. *How could we apply the learnings to the development of the trastuzumab biosimilar?* We developed a risk registry right from the start. A table was created, in which all the potential things that could go wrong were listed in column one by a cross-functional team, each providing input from their perspective. For each potential item, there was a potential cause (column two), which could have an effect (column three) on either efficacy (column four) or safety (column five). The cause-effect could impact the mechanism of action of the drug. Next, there had to be a potential solution (column six) to the potential cause, for which there had to be a mitigation plan (column seven). This risk assessment exercise was performed prior to any event occurring. The process, termed as failure mode and effect analysis, was applied to de-risk all the potential events that could lead to a failure. Jyoti led this risk analysis effort.

Rajshekhar Vanga comes across as a quiet, introverted individual. His demeanour is of one who is always in 'listening mode'. His task was to build a strong regulatory team to support global filings of the biosimilars pipeline. He was well versed with the laws and regulations involved in drug development and approval of biologics at the US FDA. At Biocon he was responsible for authoring the manufacturing processes of the trastuzumab filing. This process required close interactions with the R&D, analytical, manufacturing and quality teams, each of which wrote reports on the work they performed. Reviewing these reports and then writing the story of the entire process was a formidable task. Raj and his team delivered the nearly 2,00,000-page document. Introvert? Not at all. He had excellent communication and project management skills, which were required to compile this 'piece of art'.

The culture team

The culture of a company can be an abstract concept. To make it tangible, we created a 'culture team'. Kriti Shukla, Anita Fernandez, Akansh Dixit, Lavanya Rao,

Arindam Guha and Dharani Prasad were members of this team. They called themselves Sly5. They were critical in understanding what it takes to motivate employees to participate in activities in the department. The activities included scientific forums, cells on scientific topics, a flea market and a talent show at the end of the year. Teams started practising for this show months in advance. There were dance performances, a play, music and stand-up acts. It was always a thumping success.

The culture of an organization is built on a strong foundation of leadership, company values and commitment. Companies go through successes and failures. *What are the lessons I learnt from the failures?*

1. Anticipate risks.
2. Continuously seek novel solutions to problems and the risks identified.
3. Dig deep into a subject to find things that are not obvious.
4. Consider different ways of executing a project and make informed decisions.
5. Make a safe working environment.
6. Engage your talent. Everyone brings a unique contribution to the project. Articulate the needs of the project and assign responsibilities.
7. Create a culture by studying, listening and implementing processes.

Final thoughts on talent

Biocon had the appropriate talent, and the culture of the organization was collaborative, supportive and team-oriented. The organizational structure of R&D followed the traditional chevron of drug development, which included process sciences for drug substance and drug product, analytical sciences, bioanalytical sciences and animal sciences. The leads of each department had two full-time jobs. One to lead the function, and the other to lead a product. The organizational structure had grown organically. As the company initiated new projects, the same people took on new responsibilities. It was time for a deep review of the organization and a change.

The decision was made to develop an organizational structure based on projects and not on functions. This entailed a huge change in the responsibilities of each individual. No one had 'two jobs'. The structure comprised approximately four project groups, and each group had a portfolio of projects. The head of each group was responsible for ensuring the resourcing, timelines and innovation required for the projects. The structure was amenable to expansion, such that more projects resulted in more groups being recruited.

The restructuring was not easy to design and even more difficult to implement. A detailed process was established to communicate the complex change. Time will tell if this major shift in the organizational structure will yield efficiency in prioritization and workflow. For my part, I was supported by the human resources team of Dola Mukherjee, Arijit Das and Srija Chakraborty. The entire staff of the R&D division played a crucial role in the acceptance of this change, a testimony to the culture of collaboration and common purpose in the division.

The book would have ended here, but now there is another chapter.

A Vaccine for COVID-19

Exponential learnings of drug development in society.

March 2020. We are living in unprecedented times. There is the ever-present fear of the unknown. SARS-COV2 is causing havoc. There are no drugs to cure the disease caused by it and no vaccine to protect us from infection. Our immune system is our only weapon. I have spent my entire career studying the interactions of pathogens and the immune system. I will attempt to simplify the workings of the immune system and how it interacts with the virus. I also provide my thoughts on what are the factors that will be required for safe and effective vaccines. *Will the vaccine be the final solution for controlling this pandemic?*

I landed in the US from Bangalore on 15 March 2020, just days before the epidemic was to explode in the country. There was an eerie calm at the airport in Philadelphia.

The few people there avoided each other and did not even make eye contact, as if the virus could be transmitted just by looking at one another. I was entering a pandemic situation as an expert and as a student of immunovirology, and specifically of vaccine development for viruses. I was placed in a wonderful position where I could significantly contribute to the understanding of the science of this virus.

I went straight home from the airport. My daughter had filled the refrigerator and the pantry with all the food that I would need for the next three weeks. For home was where I would remain. Cafés and stores in the neighbourhood were all closed. People were practicing social distancing. Spring was in the air, the dogwood trees were blooming with bright pink flowers, the forsythias exploding with yellow blossoms. But there were very few people walking around in the parks. Life did not look normal. Every day of the three weeks that I was confined at home, I could not help being reminded of the Holocaust movie, *The Pianist*, where the protagonist walks through a deserted city, where he could be captured and killed at any instant. This terror is what the virus has done to us. Made us fearful of the future.

In the three weeks I spent at home, I gathered an enormous amount of information about the virus, the mechanism of the disease progression and the potential drugs that could be used to fight it. I had many online meetings with my colleagues, friends and family to collect this information.* I was invited

---

* I shared this information in several presentations, such as this one: https:// www.youtube.com/watch?v=0hcd7jhQGbU

to be part of a panel on the COVID-19 task force of the Department of Biotechnology in India, as part of an initiative to advise the leadership in the Indian Council of Medical Research on potential drugs and immunotherapies that could be tested and used to treat the disease. I shared my learnings with friends, family, students and peers, and developed a better understanding of the virus and its mechanism of pathology. This process gave me some sense of control and the motivation to share what I was learning.

About four months after the pandemic started in Wuhan, China, more than two million people were infected and more than 1,30,000 deaths were reported. Life on earth would not be the same again. A virus has destroyed the way we live and has made us, as a society, reflect on how we can ever come back to a 'normal state'.

Within weeks there were hundreds of papers flooding the different forms of media, including peer-reviewed journals, un-reviewed preliminary observations and commentary blogs on various platforms. And yet, there was, and continues to be, a limited understanding of how the virus acts in our bodies and causes havoc, and why some people can eliminate the virus and others succumb. The exponential learnings have resulted in collecting information on the biology of this virus at a pace like never before. New findings are being published every day.

The virus is transmitted through droplets small and big. These droplets enter the lung and infect the epithelial cells.

The virus is made up of an envelope and contains five proteins: spike (S), membrane (M), envelope (E), nucleocapsid (N) and hemagglutinin esterase (HE). These and twenty-six other proteins are encoded by a viral RNA molecule. Coronavirus 2 (CoV2), so named since the spike proteins resemble a crown or 'corona', is a family of viruses that infect various animals including bats, camels, birds and pigs. RNA sequence analysis was used to trace the origin of this virus, and it was implicated to be a mutation of the bat coronavirus.

Outside the cell, the virus cannot replicate, but it remains 'alive'. It is very stable. It can be dissolved by detergents. Hence handwashing is an extremely important method to prevent infection.

The virus enters the lung cells by binding of the spike protein to a protein on the cell wall (receptor) named acetylcholine esterase 2 (ACE2). A protein-digesting enzyme (called PMPRSS2) on the cell surface then breaks the spike molecules into two halves (S1 and S2). This cleavage is necessary for the fusion of the membrane of the virus with the cell wall. Once this fusion occurs, the virus injects its RNA genome into the cells. This event initiates replication. This is a highly efficient process that results in hundreds of viral particles being made by each cell. The virus quickly spreads throughout the body, since the ACE2 and TRMPSS2 receptors are expressed on many cells including those of the colon, heart and muscles.

The lifecycle of the virus and disease

PROGRESSION OF COVID-19 DISEASE

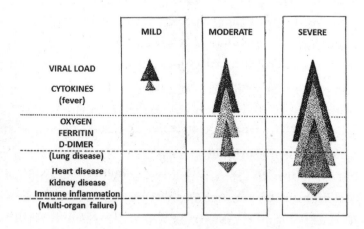

To counter the virus attack, the immune system mounts a massive immune response, activating various components of the 'armed forces'. We can use the analogy of war to understand this response. The border forces (innate immunity, antigen-presenting cells) recognize the patterns of the pathogen and inform the 'general of the immune force'—the command centre of the immune system (the CD4 T cells). The 'police' (regulatory T cells) who are responsible for surveillance, also inform the general that the virus is a bad element and needs to be destroyed. These signals enable the general to order the air force (B cells, which secrete antibodies) and army (cytotoxic T cells, which kill virus-infected cells in 'hand-to-hand' combat) to attack.

The effector cells of the immune system (T and B cells) track and follow virus-infected cells throughout the body from the lung to the heart, kidney, colon and other organs. The brain does not seem to be affected directly, but by inflammatory proteins (such as interleukin 1 and interleukin 6) secreted by the immune cells. The entire body turns into a battlefield, with hundreds of thousands of virus particles killing cells expressing the ACE2/TMPRSS2 receptor through the replication process, and a hyperactive immune system attacking all the cells in the body that are infected with the virus. Both virus and the immune system unleash an inflammatory response. The clinical term is a cytokine storm. There is death everywhere when ultimately all organs start failing, and the patient dies of either heart or lung complications due to acute respiratory distress syndrome. Patients struggle to breathe. Infection can also induce the formation of blood clots, leading to heart attacks. Autopsies of lungs of patients show the lungs filled with fluid and mucus, which destroy the lungs. All this pathology happens within days of the initial infection. The only 'hope' is that this lethal response happens in about 5 per cent of the people who are infected. Sadly, I have lost a few very good friends to this virus. Anjali Saraf, PhD, a scientist at the National Centre for Cell Science, Pune, and my classmate in college; Rajiv Kalraiyya's brother, a doctor in England, Tanaya Surve's father in Kolhapur.

About 95 per cent of the infected individuals are able to mount an immune response that clears the virus. The immune system first generates a primary response characterized by IgM antibodies to the virus, and then a secondary response of IgG antibodies. This two-step process ensures that the immune system does not mistakenly develop the wrong kind of response, such as an autoimmune response. The IgG response is much stronger, defined by amount, affinity and types of IgG antibodies. These antibodies very efficiently clear the circulating virus. The T cells, i.e., the army division of the immune system, also play a critical role in the protective immune response. These T cells secrete proteins called cytokines and chemokines, which shift the balance of the immune system from a destructive one to a protective one. Just like everything else in life, activation of the immune system is regulated by a delicate balance, which can tilt either way (destroy or protect) based on many factors, especially the overall health of an individual.

The kinetics of the immune response

PATHOGENESIS OF COVID-19

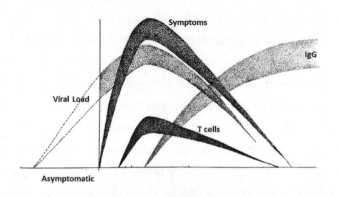

The typical symptoms occur after four to seven days of infection. During this time, the virus is happily replicating, unbeknownst to the host. If one is exposed to an infected patient, there is no escape, other than social distancing. This period of asymptomatic infection is when the virus transmits to unsuspecting hosts. Symptoms initiate with cough and fever, and some patients have difficulty breathing a little later as the disease progresses. Curiously, many patients lose the sense of smell and taste, speculated to be caused by the virus infecting the nerve endings of the nose. Children appear to be less affected, although they carry and transmit the virus. A small number of children present with a rare inflammatory condition, called MIS-C or COVID-induced multi-system inflammatory syndrome in children. The virus seems to attack almost every part of the body with a ferocity that is literally breathtaking. And we do not have a clear understanding of how the virus rampages through our body. There is no light at the end of the tunnel.

So what can we learn from the past? The 1918 influenza epidemic infected 500 million people and killed 50 million. There was no treatment and no vaccine at that time. More than a century later we still do not have a universal vaccine against the influenza virus. The virus changes its DNA, to escape the immune system; these changes (mutations) occur in two major proteins—haemagglutinin (H) and neuraminidase (N) every year. The World Health Organization predicts the strain for each year, and vaccine companies make a vaccine for that year! H3N2 is the 2019–20 strain. H1N1 was very pathogenic. These vaccines are made in chicken eggs. They are not easy to make. The influenza virus also enters the cells by a similar process as CoV2. A binding event, cleavage of the viral proteins, and then cell fusion. A universal vaccine that blocks the binding and fusion process of influenza is yet to be developed. Many institutions and industries have been attempting to do so for decades. A warning for the developers of a vaccine against CoV2 is that it will not be simple to make one that induces a neutralizing antibody to the virus. This learning is important not just from research into influenza, but into HIV. HIV also utilizes the binding and fusion process of entry. Here too, we have been unable to make a vaccine that induces broadly neutralizing antibodies that block the entry of all strains of the virus. This is one of the holy grails of the vaccine community.

It was not so long ago when we were focused on the most devastating of viruses, HIV. More than thirty years of development of the vaccine against HIV has not yielded a successful outcome. *What are the similarities and differences between HIV and coronavirus that we can learn from?* One of the major differences between the two viruses is that HIV attacks (binds and kills) the CD4 T cells (the general of the army), crippling the immune system at its heart. At least as we currently know, CoV2 does not infect any major cells of the immune system. Both viruses utilize the bind-to-receptor, proteolytic cleavage of the envelope protein, and fusion-to-host-cell membrane process to infect cells.

A successful vaccine against CoV2 should block the bind, cleave and fuse processes. We shall evaluate the strategy for developing such a vaccine later. First, there is another consideration.

The process of developing a vaccine against HIV has taught us that overall protective immunity against HIV may require both neutralizing antibodies (the air force) and the army (CD8 T cells). T cells do not recognize antigens (portions of proteins) directly, but only when they are presented to them by specialized molecules called major histocompatibility complex (MHC) proteins. CD8 T cells recognize antigens presented by MHC-I, and CD4 T cells by MHC-II. For CD8 T cells to develop into killer cytotoxic T cells (CTL), they must be activated by an antigen presented through an intracellular antigen presenting pathway. In this pathway, antigens must be expressed from genes in the nucleus of the cell. CD4 T cells develop into helper cells upon being stimulated by extracellular antigens. Once activated, CD4 T cells provide helper signals (such as soluble activating proteins called cytokines) to activate CD8 T cells. These CD8 CTL hunt down virus-infected cells and kill the cells and the virus in it. This arm of the immune system is called the cell-mediated immune response. Should a vaccine induce this arm of the immune response for it to be effective? How is the CD8 T cell protective response induced by a vaccine? We will evaluate some of these considerations in the design of a vaccine for COVID-19.

First, let us understand the vastness of the problem. There are hundreds of thousands of people who are falling extremely sick, of which approximately 4 per cent are dying; millions of people are exposed and diagnosed; millions more are exposed and not diagnosed; billions of people need to be vaccinated. These numbers underscore the challenge for humanity, which is one like never before. *So what is it going to take to vaccinate the planet against this coronavirus?* During a process of developing a vaccine, a target product profile (TPP) is first generated. This TPP process defines the requirements, against which the vaccine can be designed and produced. The table below lists the considerations for designing the vaccine.

Target product profile

Vaccine characteristics	Requirements
Indication for use	Prevention of infection Control of disease progression, if infected
Contraindication	Should not affect responses to other vaccines
Target population	Healthcare workers and contacts and the entire population of the world
Safety/Reactogenicity	Should not induce any major side effects
Measures of efficacy	Generates antibodies that block entry of the virus Activates cytotoxic T cells
Dose regimen	One or two doses
Durability of protection	At least one to two years
Route of administration	Subcutaneous
Product stability and storage	Should be stable at room temperature for at least two weeks

The virus contains several proteins: S, M, E, NE. Which of these proteins is the best target for developing an effective vaccine? In the course of developing vaccines over the years, we have learnt that identifying the dominant antigen that will induce a protective immune response is not straightforward. Most viruses utilize more than one protein to enter and fuse with cells. Human papilloma virus utilizes L1 and L2, influenza utilizes hemagglutinin and neuraminidase, and HIV requires gp120 and gp41. Viruses have evolved over millions of years to trick the immune system and invade the body by escaping the immune attack. The immune system has to evoke an equal and opposite reaction to the replicative potential of the virus. To do this, the immune system must expand exponentially and attack the virus-infected cells violently. This violent immune attack is one of the causes of the rapid progression of this disease, which leads to death just days after the infection.

An optimal vaccine should induce neutralizing antibodies that block the entry and fusion processes of the virus. In addition, a cytotoxic T cell response may be required to effectively kill virus-infected cells, in the event the virus escapes the antibody blockade. It sounds fairly straightforward, but in normal times, it takes ten to twenty years to develop a vaccine. *Why does it take so long?*

The process of vaccine development

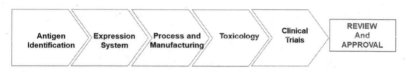

Developing a vaccine is a multistep process, each taking months or even years of research and preparation. Step one entails identifying the region of the virus that can elicit the protective immune response. Fortunately, scientists have done this work and the experiments suggest that antibodies directed at the spike protein can block viral entry into cells.

Step two involves delivering the spike protein in the appropriate conformation. Very high magnification crystal structure studies of the spike protein and the entry process have demonstrated that the trimer-structure (i.e., three proteins come together) of the spike protein is required for entry. Based on this observation, the spike protein that needs to be expressed in the patients must express the trimer structure. Furthermore, to induce activation of CD8 T cells, the spike protein needs to be expressed through an intracellular expression process. There are several platforms to express the spike protein. The table below shows the various approaches, and the likelihood of activation of CD4 (antibody) and CD8 (CTL) responses.

	CD4 (humoral)	CD8 (CMI)	Potential safety
DNA	+	+	+++
RNA	+	+	+++
Protein	+	-	++++
Viral vector	++	++	++
Inactivated virus	++++	-	++
Attenuated live virus	+++++	+++++	+

Step three entails developing a scalable process to manufacture the vaccine in large amounts. Even if we consider only healthcare workers and healthy contacts, at least one to two billion doses of the vaccine will need to be manufactured. The manufacturing process is dependent on the platforms listed above. As an example, a viral vector manufacturing facility requires the following steps:

1. Engineering the viral vector to insert the CoV2 spike gene.
2. Growing the virus vector in cells by the process of fermentation (much like fermentation for beer). This process is termed an upstream process, where the cells are grown in large fermenters.
3. After the fermentation process has been completed, viral vector particles must be purified from several thousand litres of culture media. All impurities associated with the cells, the growth media, etc., need to be separated through processes of chromatography. This process is termed as the downstream process. The bulk viral vector then needs to be transferred into vials, which then can be used for safety toxicology studies and clinical trials.

All these processes are highly regulated by GMP. The processes need to be extensively characterized and validated for consistency and accuracy to ensure that each batch of the vaccine is able to induce the required protective immune response. All the processes above are monitored closely by a battery of analytical methods.

Step four is conducting toxicology studies. The vaccine product must be tested for toxicity in animals. This is an intensive study of all the potential side effects a vaccine may induce, prior to administration to humans. A maximum tolerated dose is determined through these processes. These studies are also highly regulated by both regulatory bodies as well as ethics committees.

Step five involves clinical trials. Clinical research is initiated in phase one studies, which are smaller studies designed to ensure the vaccine is safe. Phase two trials are designed to test the hypothesis that the vaccine will induce a sufficient protective immune response. Safety end points continue to be measures. Finally, phase three trials are performed to provide definitive evidence of the efficacy and safety of the vaccine. For this purpose, double-blind trials are performed, where neither the recipient nor the person administering the vaccine know whether the individual is receiving the vaccine or a placebo. All trials are done under the regulations of regulatory bodies and ethics and safety committees. Subjects are given information about the risks of the vaccine and participate in the study only after informed consent.

Step six entails regulatory review and approval. After the phase three trial is completed, the data sets of the manufacturing process, toxicology studies and clinical trials are submitted to the appropriate agencies. A review of these documents and an audit of the facilities that manufacture the vaccine are conducted.

Step seven is approval of the vaccine. If all the predefined criteria of efficacy and safety of the vaccine are met, and the manufacturing facility and processes are duly audited, then the agency approves the commercialization of the vaccine.

As you can see, developing a vaccine is no trivial task. It is a long and arduous process. For COVID-19, this process had to be accelerated in an unprecedented manner. *How was this achieved?*

Generally, a company or academic institution that is involved in vaccine development has the expertise and capabilities to develop a vaccine by means of one or two of the possible processes. Hence, each institution develops the vaccine they have expertise in. In the case of CoV2, a systematic comparison of all approaches to making a vaccine that would induce the appropriate immune response was needed. The collaboration required academia, industry, governments, regulatory bodies and philanthropic organizations to come together.

December 2020. It is a remarkable time in the history of drug development. The data to demonstrate the efficacy and safety of the first vaccine for COVID-19 is about to be presented to the advisory committee of the FDA. Live. On TV. Linny Vinny, who has become a good friend over the past six months and has been coming to my house every other week to help me 'keep it clean', is with me. Linny and I have been discussing many issues about the science of the pandemic for months. On 7 December, at 9 a.m., I put on CNBC TV and watch the proceedings of the FDA advisory committee. Linny says to me, 'This is your equivalent of binge-watching *The Sopranos*.' I laugh and say, 'Yes!'

The process of getting advice from a detailed review of the results of the vaccine development process is not unique to this vaccine; it is done for every novel drug that the FDA approves. And it is transparent and always done on live television.

The FDA advisory committee comprises several well-known and accomplished scientists, clinicians, academics, government personnel, an army doctor and Paul Offit. Paul is a star in the vaccine world. He has so much experience, and I revere his opinion. The programme starts with the FDA moderator, Dr Prabha Attrey, announcing the sequence of events for the day. It will be a nine-hour marathon review. I am prepared with my notebook, chai and snacks.

The CDC representative gives an overview of the status of the pandemic. In the US, it is at a peak, as the country is just coming out of Thanksgiving and going into Christmas. There are over 1,00,000 cases a day, and over 5000 COVID-related deaths a day. Shocking. The FDA director announces that since Congress and the President have declared that the pandemic is a national emergency, the FDA is authorized to evoke an unparalleled approval process called 'emergency use approval'. This kind of approval has never been given before. Even during previous pandemics.

I almost shriek in delight when I hear that my friend and colleague, Kathrin Jansen, the head of the vaccine programme at Pfizer, is going to present the data on the mRNA vaccine that she led.

Kathrin did her PhD at the Philips University, in Marburg, Germany, and post-doctoral training at Cornell University. I worked with her very closely when she led the R&D team at Merck in the development of the HPV vaccine Gardasil. Her leadership skills, ability to empower teams to work at their highest capacity, and laser-like focus on the goal are qualities that were critical in developing this vaccine against COVID-19. I could not think of a better leader than Kathrin to deliver successfully on an almost impossible task.

On the day of the FDA advisory review, she presents in her characteristic calm, fully-in-control manner, recounting the story of the vaccine, the preclinical pharmacology, toxicology and manufacturing aspects. The head of the clinical team then presents the results of the double-blind clinical trials. The results are an astounding 95 per cent efficacy against severe infection, i.e., 95 per cent of the people who got the placebo contracted COVID-19, but only 5 per cent in the vaccinated group got the disease. The efficacy was tested three months after the second shot. The side effects of the vaccine evaluated thus far showed no major safety concerns. Local injection-site reactions were noted in several people, but these are normal for a vaccine. They indicate that the body is reacting to the vaccine, which is a good sign.

Next, there is a barrage of questions from the committee. A total of sixty-five questions are asked over the course of five hours. Some of the questions were:

- How will you measure asymptomatic infections?
- Does the mRNA activate TLR7/8 and induce innate immune responses?
- Did you observe any allergic responses?
- How quickly is the mRNA salvaged; does it activate endogenous retroviruses?
- Did you examine the viral sequences in the eight subjects in the vaccine group that got infected?
- Aren't 162 subjects out of 30,000 a much lower incidence?
- Did you follow up with some individuals for more than four months?
- How sure are you that antibody responses confer protection?
- Is the effect in sixteen- to seventeen-year-olds different? Is extrapolation possible?
- The number of volunteers for trials in race/ethnicity are low; will this be increased?

Finally, after a gruelling question and answer session, it is time to vote. On live television. The FDA moderator asks the question, 'Based on the totality of the evidence available, do the benefits of the Pfizer-BioNTech COVID-19 vaccine outweigh its risks for use in individuals sixteen years of age and older?' The results are seventeen yeses, four noes, and one abstention. After the vote, each person explains why they had voted as they did. The major concern among those who had voted 'no' seemed to be administering the vaccine to individuals younger than eighteen years, since the trial was done in those over eighteen years old. There were other concerns, but the FDA gave emergency use approval within forty-eight hours of the advisory committee review. The race was now on to administer the vaccine to millions, if not billions, of people.

On 17 December 2020, Moderna presented the results of its mRNA vaccine to the FDA advisory committee. Jacqueline Miller, a friend from my Merck days, presented the results of the clinical trial. Jackie had trained at the University of Pennsylvania as a nephrologist. She went on to work at Merck Vaccines, and had extraordinary experience in developing the rotavirus vaccine and later the chicken pox shingles vaccine when she moved to GSK. In February 2020, she was recruited to Moderna to lead the clinical development programme for the COVID-19 vaccine. It was an opportunity of a lifetime to develop a vaccine to 'save the world' from the pandemic.

The bar was higher than that for the Pfizer vaccine. There were new mutations of the virus circulating in the population. The Brazil strain (P.1), the South Africa strain (B.1.351), the British strain (B.1.1.7). The vaccine needed to protect individuals against all the strains. Would the data be sufficient to convince the review committee? It was. Moderna got a 16:0 vote in favour of approval. It was an amazing review and results. Again, I sat and watched the nine-hour presentation with rapt attention.

The Moderna vaccine was also granted emergency use approval by the FDA.

And on 8 March 2021, Johnson & Johnson's adenovirus-26-based vaccine was also granted emergency use approval, again with a 16:0 vote. This is a single-dose vaccine, which is stable in the fridge. The previous two vaccines needed to be kept frozen at -70°C (Pfizer) and -20°C (Moderna). Maintaining an unbroken cold chain was a major challenge for widespread supply and distribution.

As of August 2021, more than a billion people have been vaccinated. We are approaching herd immunity. When will life be 'normal' again? Maybe never. And that is okay. We are transitioning from deep winter and are back to a beautiful spring in Philadelphia.

In spite of the unprecedented speed with which the vaccines against COVID-19 were developed, the story of the pandemic is evolving rapidly every month, every day, it seems. New mutants are emerging. A million sequences of the virus are now reported on the website that has been collecting this information (https://nextstrain.org/ncov/global). However, fortunately, at least for now, several studies are reporting that the major mutant strains in different geographies are still being blocked by antibodies induced by the vaccines in the majority of individuals. Some breakthrough cases, that is, people getting infected despite being vaccinated, are also being published in high profile journals such as the *New England Journal of Medicine* and *Nature*. Again, these breakthrough cases are rare.

India is on fire (approximately 3,00,000 cases are being reported a day). The potential reasons behind this huge surge are that firstly, between January and March 2021, there was no lockdown. People attended parties and weddings, election rallies were held, as was the Kumbh Mela. This people-to-people interaction may have resulted in extensive spread of the virus. Secondly, the virus has mutated. There are four major strains circulating, and some of the mutants have been reported to be highly infectious and replicate more efficiently. Thirdly, a highly active immune system in people (due to several previous secondary infections) makes them more susceptible to infection. Fourth is the un(hygiene) hypothesis. People who have had exposure to other infections can have a heightened baseline inflammatory response, which can result in a more aggressive form of COVID-19 infection. Fifth is the lack of an efficient vaccine supply and distribution system. Sixth is a lack of awareness about the importance of a mask or exhaustion with regard to the use of masks. Seventh is better and a more accurate reporting of cases and deaths.

The multifactorial causes of the exponential increase in viral spread in India are perplexing scientists the world over. There is no one answer. Time will tell the real story of this pandemic.

Until then, we have to wait and see.

Epilogue

The stories of the failures and success of various drugs that I have narrated are my observations and interpretations of the so many aspects involved. The people in the stories, to me, are the most important. Their dedication and passion have been such an important part of the journey.

The exponential learnings from the **vaccines** such as Rotavirus and HIV among many others enabled the world to witness the development the COVID-19 vaccines in unprecedented timelines. This accomplishment would not have been possible without extensive collaboration, and most importantly a sense of common purpose.

Immune therapies of cancer by the immune checkpoint inhibitors have resulted from decades of progressive learnings of many, many molecules, pathways, and signal transduction cascades. These successes (that are only possible by standing on the shoulders of giants!) culminated in discoveries which harness the power of the immune system to kill cancer cells.

Cell therapies, which are revolutionizing the treatment of various leukaemias dare we say curing some of them. Newer design of CAR-T cells will enable larger and larger groups of patients and cancers to be treated.

Gene therapy, one of the final frontiers of therapy, which underwent through a lot of sequential failure, has finally seen some success stories with treatments for certain types of blindness and muscular dystrophies.

I started by discussing Murali's living-with-haemophilia. I end the book with the story I started with, about my best friend, Murali. Murali has a mutation in a few nucleotides in a gene that encodes for the protein factor VIII, the absence of which prevents blood from clotting. Administering the normal gene to Murali should be able to correct his disease. After learning so many aspects of drug development, are we ready to find a cure for genetic defects like Murali's? Yes. We are very close.

With the success of gene therapy in treating rare diseases of the eye and muscle, there is a glimmer of hope for Murali, who could benefit greatly from this therapy for haemophilia. Physician-scientists Kathrine High in Philadelphia and Anil Nathwani in London have been working on developing gene therapy for the treatment of haemophilia for over twenty years. There have been several clinical trials using various viral vectors, including adenoviruses and adeno-associated viruses. So far, none of the potential therapies has been able to successfully cure/ treat the disease. The immune response that is generated to the vector and the 'normal' factor in these patients eliminates the protein. These are extremely difficult clinical studies to perform.

BioMarin, a biotechnology company based in San Rafael, California, has been conducting clinical trials to treat haemophilia using AAV vectors. The product is called valoctocogene roxaparvovec and the results of the trials are encouraging.[*] The approval of this drug is now eagerly awaited by the haemophilia community. But we will have to wait until the safety and efficacy of the drug are clearly established. The light at the end of the gene therapy tunnel is now seen as a flicker. The availability of a gene therapy drug to treat haemophilia will be a landmark event in the history of treatment of diseases.

As for me, I have started all over again. With my friend of forty-five years, Ravi Khare, I have ventured into the world of data analytics. Ravi has decades of experience in the fields of engineering, mathematics and statistics, while I have deep experience in biology and medicines. We are combining our knowledge to find 'engineering solutions to solve biological problems'. What inflection points we will

---

[*] Pasi, K.J., Rangarajan, S., Mitchell, N., Lester, W., Symington, E., Madan, B., Laffan, M., Russell, C.B., Li, M., Pierce, G.F. and Wong, W.Y. 'Multiyear Follow-up of AAV5-hFVIII-SQ Gene Therapy for Hemophilia A'. *New England Journal of Medicine* 382 (2020): 29–40.

need to find these solutions, only time will tell. We are focused on the journey, taking on tough projects.

I have been blessed with the opportunity to work on many journeys of both failures and successes. Writing this book has been my attempt to make sense of the learnings and share my experience and knowledge to help develop affordable and high-quality drugs for mankind.

Acknowledgements

This book is an autobiographical documentation of my experiences in drug development. Writing this book has been on my mind for many years, but required my retiring from my corporate life. It has taken me more than two years to write this book, talking to and interviewing my friends and colleagues, some of whom I have mentioned in the various chapters. I have enjoyed writing this book in planes, trains and automobiles in my travels. I 'remembered' so many small incidents and anecdotes through these conversations. My immediate and extended family has been my rock-solid support during my journey. Preeti, Anjali, Shyamala, Ujjwala, Ravi, Manohar and Ajit (this generation); Anisha, Lin, Dipti, Vikram, Kshamta, Jaideep and Ranjit (next-gen). Murali, my dear friend, has helped me by talking through various ideas every week at 2.15 p.m., while he has his lunch. Kavitha Iyer-Rodrigues, Jacqueline Miller, Vijay Chandru, Bruce Levine, Madhu Dikshit, Siddhartha Mukherjee and Paul Offit for reading the proofs and Gauri Divate for the beautifully done artwork. Gurveen Chadha, my editor, who supported the idea and concept of describing failures, has been a constant force that kept me on track. Finally, the conversations of many students who have attended the sessions of the 'regulatory aspects of drug-development' course, which crystallized the stories of each failure. Will there be a follow-up book? Yes, but maybe after I get some feedback on this one.